EDUCATING NURSES

EDUCATING NURSES

A Call for Radical Transformation

Patricia Benner

Molly Sutphen

Victoria Leonard

Lisa Day

○

Foreword by
Lee S. Shulman

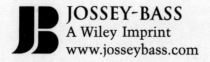

JOSSEY-BASS
A Wiley Imprint
www.josseybass.com

Published by Jossey-Bass
A Wiley Imprint
989 Market Street, San Francisco, CA 94103-1741—www.josseybass.com

Readers should be aware that Internet Web sites offered as citations and/or sources for further information may have changed or disappeared between the time this was written and when it is read.

Jossey-Bass books and products are available through most bookstores. To contact Jossey-Bass directly call our Customer Care Department within the U.S. at 800-956-7739, outside the U.S. at 317-572-3986, or fax 317-572-4002.

Jossey-Bass also publishes its books in a variety of electronic formats. Some content that appears in print may not be available in electronic books.

Library of Congress Cataloging-in-Publication Data

Educating nurses : a call for radical transformation / Patricia Benner ... [et al.] ; foreword by Lee S. Shulman. – 1st ed.
p. ; cm. – (Jossey-Bass higher and adult education series) (Preparation for the professions series)
Includes bibliographical references and index.
ISBN 978-0-470-45796-2 (cloth)
1. Nursing – Study and teaching. I. Benner, Patricia E. II. Series: Jossey-Bass higher and adult education series. III. Series: Preparation for the professions series.
[DNLM: 1. Education, Nursing–trends. WY 18 E235 2010]   RT73.E38 2010
610.73076–dc22

                 2009031936

Printed in the United States of America
FIRST EDITION
HB Printing 15 14 13 12

The Jossey-Bass
Higher and Adult Education Series

THE PREPARATION FOR THE PROFESSIONS SERIES

THE PREPARATION for the Professions Series reports the results of the Carnegie Foundation for the Advancement of Teaching's Preparation for the Professions Program, a comparative study of professional education in medicine, nursing, law, engineering, and preparation of the clergy.

CONTENTS

FOREWORD

SOME WORDS ARE regularly misspelled. Among them is the word *foreword*, often spelled *forward*. The pages that follow are not intended to look forward beyond the narrative, argument, findings, and recommendations of this volume on the preparation of nurses. They are intended as a set of reflections that come "before the word," as antecedent to the texts that constitute the heart of this book. Forewords are appetizers rather than main courses. Indeed, they are not even that substantial; perhaps they can be compared to the bite-size *amuse-bouche* that chefs present before a meal as a small conceit to remind the patrons that there's a serious cook in the kitchen. Its intent is to amuse or tickle the tongue but also as a subtle communication, a wink from the kitchen. Shall we think of the foreword as an *amuse-pensee* or even as an *amuse-esprit*?

Ironically, the foreword is typically the *last* piece of text composed for a book and nearly always by someone who is not among the authors. Although it is the first word to be read, it is the last to be written. So it is on this occasion. Indeed, I prepare this Foreword looking back not only on the Carnegie studies of nursing education, but on the full series of Carnegie's program on preparation for the professions that took place over more than a decade. Law and engineering, the rabbinate, priesthood and ministry, medicine and nursing, school teaching and university professing, all were objects of inquiry and deliberation, of data gathering and analysis, of investigations and convenings, within and beyond the Carnegie Foundation's hillside home.

From my vantage point in the kitchen, I take this occasion to reflect on our studies of nursing education through the lens of all the other studies we conducted during the past decade. What is particularly striking is the extent to which nursing is a hybrid, a profession whose distinctive features mirror many of the central attributes of other professions while also creating a singular identity of its own. Indeed, when I look at the work of nurses, I see reflections of each of the other professions we have studied.

I will never forget the response we received from a group of nurses in North Carolina when we asked, "What is a nurse?" Their response: "As a nurse, I am the patient's last line of defense." No other conception of the nurse's role prevailed in our interviews and observations as much as the role of the nurse as patient advocate, that last line of defense against the impersonal nature of the health care system. Repeatedly we heard nurses, nursing students, and nursing faculty refer to "patient advocate" as the central role of the nurse, the heart of nursing identity. As we came to appreciate in our studies of legal education, advocacy is no simple concept. It is more than defending the rights of the client; there are times when clients must face their responsibilities and obligations, not merely defend their rights. What are the limits of zealous advocacy? The nurse is also a member of the health care team and shares responsibility for maintaining the quality of health care for the larger community.

As an educator, in particular as an educator of teachers, I was equally struck by the attention to the role of nurse as teacher. The work of a nurse is not complete, we were told, when a disease has been healed but when a patient has been prepared to return to a life that is self-managed and independent. For this nurses regularly are expected to teach: to explain to patients how they must care for themselves and why, what new habits of eating and exercising, self-examination and self-regulation they need to develop in order to live healthy productive lives. Who teaches? Nurses teach.

One need only spend a few hours with nurses on a hospital floor or in a cancer treatment room, in an individual office or even during a home visit, before being struck by the varieties of technology with which the nurse must competently cope. Some technologies are as exotic as the now-typical arrays of sensing devices in an ICU or the daunting devices needed for dialysis. Others appear as pedestrian as a hypodermic syringe or a blood pressure cuff. And computers are ubiquitous for record keeping, communications, and the monitoring of drugs. All these now fall within the nurse's responsibilities, and he or she is expected to understand what and how to perform in those circumstances. There is an element of engineering and technology in that role, as much *Star Trek* as *ER*.

The nurse "ministers" to patients; he or she offers care and consolation, encouragement and understanding. Much like clergy, we expect nurses to understand how to respond to pain and anxiety, to nurture patients in the face of the terror of the unknown, and to offer hope when there appears to be little available. At times, nurses act as rabbis or priests, comforting family members and caring for the ill. There is a recurring element of spirituality in that caring, even aspects of faith and dedication.

Thus when I think about the preparation of nurses, I see key elements of preparing lawyers and teachers, engineers and ministers, physicians and psychotherapists, social workers and institutional managers. The work is physically grueling and intellectually taxing. It is both routine and filled with the unexpected and the surprising. Nursing education is preparation for remarkably hard work.

This complexity and richness characteristic of the nursing profession is paralleled by the complexity of its contexts of practice. In most other professions, the practitioners maintain a certain modicum of control over the pace and density of the services they render. They normally can limit their attention to a single patient, client, case, or design at a time. But in nursing, much like teaching, many clients are present at the same time, often all needing attention and care. Some form of "batch processing" may be possible in teaching, as when a teacher instructs a large or a small group. But nursing typically requires one-on-one attention and treatment. Thus, some form of "triage" is needed on a continuing basis.

Nursing is indeed a hybrid profession, an interdisciplinary and inter-professional nexus of roles and obligations. At its core, however, remain the expectations for caring and advocacy, for ministering to the needs of those who are ill. Hybrids are often particularly robust because they combine the strengths of several species into one. But they may also be particularly vulnerable.

The historian Susan Reverby has made the poignant observation that nurses are "obliged to care" in a society that does not value caring. Not only are nurses offered little respect and only moderate financial compensation, they are also licensed to practice with less formal education than any of the other professions. While medicine, law, and the clergy generally expect post-baccalaureate preparation, and teaching and engineering require at least a bachelor's degree and often more, nurses can currently practice with only a two-year associate's degree. It is mind-boggling that this profession, this hybrid of advocacy and medicine, engineering and ministry, teaching and caring, can be practiced with less formal preparation than any other academic profession. It is a challenge that the authors of this book address directly. It will be a significant aspect of the issues and controversies that the book provokes.

When the Carnegie Foundation was ready to address the challenges of nursing education, we scoured the country for the ideal person to lead the study. One name was proposed repeatedly; she lived and worked in our backyard at the University of California San Francisco School of Nursing. Patricia Benner was a social scientist and humanist, an experienced nurse and a chaired professor; someone initially trained as a nurse at Pasadena City College who received her doctorate at Berkeley, a distinguished scholar and a conscience to her profession. We asked. Patricia agreed. We had the leader this work required.

As her alter ego, we needed someone who would bring a very different set of perspectives to the inquiry, who would serve as complement and compatriot with both research training and scholarly experience from another direction. Molly Sutphen had originally pursued studies as a physical anthropologist and anatomist until she was captured by the history of science and medicine. After completing her doctorate in the history of medicine at Yale, she continued to do research and to teach in medical schools. The opportunity to spend four years studying and writing about the preparation of nurses was irresistible to Molly and her talents were irresistible to Carnegie.

Patricia rounded out the nursing team by going to two of her own former students who were now pursuing distinguished careers as nursing educators and practitioners. Victoria Leonard, now a health consultant at the UCSF California Childcare Health Program, and Lisa Day, a clinical nurse specialist for Neuroscience and Critical Care at UCSF Medical Center, joined the team.

Finally, the work was supported by the senior scholars who had coordinated our studies of education in the professions from the very beginning—Anne Colby and William Sullivan. The former is a notable life-span developmental psychologist with special interest in the moral development of adults, and the latter is a superb philosopher/social scientist who has written extensively about "habits of the heart" and the ethical aspects of professional work. Their role was to collaborate actively in every study we conducted as well as to stitch together the separate professional education studies so they emerged as more than the sum of their parts.

This Foreword cannot do justice to the volume it introduces without acknowledging that this book indeed looks forward with wisdom, courage, and a premeditated dose of provocation to the needed reforms of the field of heath education in general and nursing education in particular. Patricia Benner has served as a beloved gadfly within the nursing community for decades, even as she has been properly admired, even venerated, for her contributions to the theory and practice of the field. This book is neither an apologetic nor a rationalization for current practice. It holds up a mirror to the field and, while applauding it for its superb accomplishments in the face of many barriers, it also is unambiguously critical of the status quo and quite specific about what remains to be done. As such, it is a worthy addition to the lineage of critical Carnegie studies, going back to Abraham Flexner's 1910 report on medical education a century ago up to the studies on law, the clergy, and engineering published recently. I applaud Patricia Benner, Molly Sutphen, Victoria Leonard, Lisa Day, and

Carnegie's entire staff for the professions programs for this superb contribution. I look forward to witnessing its impact on the field of nursing education.

I hope that your intellectual palates have been stimulated and your interest provoked. I know that personally I could not imagine being more enlightened and stimulated during the past ten years than I have been by our studies of education in the professions.

Lee S. Shulman
President Emeritus
The Carnegie Foundation for the Advancement of Teaching
Stanford, California

ACKNOWLEDGMENTS

FIRST AND FOREMOST, we wish to thank past Carnegie President Dr. Lee Shulman, who with Senior Carnegie Scholars Drs. Anne Colby and William Sullivan envisioned this large program of research Preparation of the Professions. Dr. Lee Shulman lent generous and inspiring guidance, including participating in one of our site visits and attending our research debriefing meetings throughout the project. Colby and Sullivan guided and coordinated this study with the wisdom that they had gained from the studies of clergy, engineers, lawyers, and physicians. They participated in site visits and debriefings and many nursing study group meetings. We are grateful for their keen scholarly and practical guidance. We also thank senior Carnegie scholars who conducted site visits with us: Gordon Russell (Carnegie board member), Dr. Mary Huber, Dr. Alex McCormick, Molly Cooke, M.D., Dr. David Irby, and Dr. Bridget O'Brien. Dr. Lori Rodriguez signed on at the inception of the project as a research assistant and doctoral student. She designed and completed her dissertation on teaching about practice breakdown and errors in undergraduate nursing education. Dr. Rodriguez went on all the site visits and participated in the site visit instrument development. We are also grateful for the contributions of doctoral students Dr. Liana Hain, Dr. Susan McNiesh, and Mary Nottingham. Thank you for your generous contributions to the project!

We simply could not have done this study without the enthusiastic participation of the nine participant schools of nursing, their administrators, faculty, and students, who opened their schools, classrooms, and clinical sites for us to observe and ask questions. We listened and learned from your experiences and observations. Thank you to the Samuel Merritt School of Nursing; Riverside School of Nursing; Roberts Wesleyan School of Nursing; Saddleback Community College, Department of Nursing; University of California San Francisco School of Nursing; University of North Carolina School of Nursing; University of South Dakota School of Nursing; University of Washington School of Nursing; and Villanova University School of Nursing. We appreciate the openness, hospitality, and genuine interest in the study that we encountered at all the schools.

We are also grateful to our nursing organization collaborators and partners whose counsel and support made the project better: the American Association of Colleges of Nursing, American Nurses' Association, National Council of State Boards of Nursing, National League for Nursing, and National Student Nurses' Association. In the tradition of the Carnegie Foundation for the Advancement of Teaching, we now give the study to your stewardship, along with students, nurse educators, and all stakeholders in improving nursing education to make the findings accessible and useful within the profession.

Nursing scholars and leaders were frequent and useful advisors on this project. Thank you, Dr. Pat Cross, Carnegie Foundation for the Advancement of Teaching board member and internationally known scholar in higher education, for your careful and most useful early read and critique of the manuscript. We are particularly grateful to Dr. Christine Tanner of Oregon Health Sciences University and Eloise Balasco Cathcart of New York University, who consulted with us all along the way, including reading drafts of this manuscript and making many helpful suggestions. Also many colleagues at AACN and NLN, in particular Dr. Beverly Malone and Dr. Kathy Kauffman, Dr. Pamela Ironside, and Dr. Terry Valiga at NLN; Dr. Polly Bednash, and AACN board members who reviewed the study early and late.

Dr. Ellen Wert, a gifted developmental editor, worked on all the Carnegie Studies of professional education and brought out insights and continuities among the studies at the final writing stages. Thank you, Ellen, for helping us make this research report more accessible and instructive! We had three assistants who helped at one point or another during the project: Megan Mills, Molly Romanow, and Nisha Patel each contributed talent and commitment to the project.

Last but not least, we are grateful to the Atlantic Philanthropies and the Carnegie Foundation for the Advancement of Teaching, who funded this project. The Thelma Shobe Endowed Chair in Nursing and Spirituality at the University of California, San Francisco, contributed to funding our research team and consultants. This study was a focal interest of Thelma Cook, who established and funded the Shobe Endowed Chair. Patricia Benner was the Thelma Shobe Endowed Professor at the time of the study. The Thelma Shobe Chair funded research associates at key points during the study. We are also grateful to the University of California, San Francisco, particularly our dean, Dr. Kathy Dracup, who also supported this project through donating significant portions of the research team's time, and meeting and workspaces.

Thank you all for your contributions to this work!

Patricia Benner
Molly Sutphen
Victoria Leonard
Lisa Day

THE AUTHORS

Dr. *Patricia Benner* is a senior scholar with the Carnegie Foundation for the Advancement of Teaching. She is also a professor emerita at the University of California San Francisco School of Nursing. She is a noted nursing educator and author of *From Novice to Expert: Excellence and Power in Nursing Practice*, which has been translated into eight languages. She is the director of this Carnegie Foundation for the Advancement of Teaching National Nursing Education Study, which is the first such study in forty years. Additionally, she collaborated with the Carnegie Preparation for the Professions studies of clergy, engineering, law, and medicine. Dr. Benner is a fellow of the American Academy of Nursing. She was elected an honorary fellow of the Royal College of Nursing. Her work has influence beyond nursing in the areas of clinical practice and clinical ethics. She has received two honorary doctorates. She is the first author of *Expertise in Nursing Practice: Caring, Ethics and Clinical Judgment* (2009) with Christine Tanner and Catherine Chesla, and she has coauthored twelve other notable books.

Dr. *Molly Sutphen* is a research scholar at the Carnegie Foundation for the Advancement of Teaching and co-director of the Carnegie Foundation National Nursing Education Study. She is also an assistant adjunct professor in the Department of Social and Behavioral Sciences at the University of California, San Francisco. She is a historian of public health, medicine, and nursing. She has taught history, ethics, and global health to medical, pharmacy, and nursing students at the University of California, San Francisco. She has published numerous articles on nursing education and the history of public health and is finishing the book *An Imperial Hygenist*. She received her doctorate from Yale University in the history of medicine and the life sciences.

Victoria Leonard is a family nurse practitioner and child care health consultant at the University of California San Francisco (UCSF) California Childcare Health Program. She is a trainer for Child Care Health Consultants in California and does trainings and presentations, as well as writing educational materials on health and safety issues for child care providers in the state. She has taught health policy and ethics and pediatrics in the nurse practitioner program at UCSF and has worked with children and families with chronic illnesses in pediatric subspecialty clinics. Leonard was a research associate for the Carnegie Foundation National Nursing Education Study and participated in the data collection, analysis, and writing up of the findings. She has also consulted on a longitudinal research study of teen mothers and their infants for the past fifteen years. She received her Ph.D. from the UCSF School of Nursing.

Lisa Day graduated from Long Beach City College in California with an associate degree in nursing in 1984. She has worked as a nurse in a postanesthesia recovery room, a medical cardiac intensive care unit, and a neuroscience critical care unit, and she completed her B.S.N, M.S., and Ph.D. (with Patricia Benner) at the University of California San Francisco School of Nursing. She taught prelicensure nursing in an accelerated second degree program for eight years before recently returning to clinical practice; she is now the clinical nurse specialist for neuroscience and critical care at UCSF Medical Center. Day has been involved as a consultant in several projects related to nursing education, including the RWJ-funded Quality and Safety Education in Nursing (QSEN), the Helene Fuld Health Trust–funded project Evaluating the Outcomes of Accelerated Nursing Education, and evaluation of the Oregon Consortium for Nursing Education (OCNE); and she participated in the 2008 National League for Nursing think tank on Transforming Clinical Nursing Education.

EDUCATING NURSES

INTRODUCTION

THE PROFESSION OF nursing in the United States is at a significant moment. Profound changes in science, technology, patient activism, the market-driven health care environment, and the nature and settings of nursing practice have all radically transformed nursing practice since the last national nursing education study, almost forty years ago (Lysaught, 1970). The changes in nursing practice, in turn, have enormous implications for nursing education.

Indeed, a list of just a few of the changes in nursing practice suggests many implications for nursing education. Nurses now do most bedside monitoring, make almost all home visits, assist and teach aging patients to manage multiple chronic illnesses, and deliver much of everyday primary care. Nurses maintain patient safety while managing multiple intrusive technologies where the margin of error is extremely narrow, and they do so in increasingly complex, hazardous work environments. Nurses administer care in widely diverse settings, ranging from specialized acute hospital bedside care to in-home and long-term nursing care for the technologically dependent and aging, as well as school and community nursing care. Although charged with caring for patients with increasingly complicated diagnostic and treatment regimes in hospital settings, nurses may also deliver care to patients with similar needs in ambulatory settings, the community, and the home.

New nurses need to be prepared to practice safely, accurately, and compassionately, in varied settings, where knowledge and innovation increase at an astonishing rate. They must enter practice ready to continue learning, often through self-directed learning that can be adapted to any site of practice, from school nursing to intensive care nursing. To practice safely and effectively, today's new nurses must understand a range of nursing knowledge and science, from normal and pathological physiology to genomics, pharmacology, biochemical implications of laboratory medicine for the patient's therapies, the physics of gas exchange in the lungs, cell-level transport of oxygen for the acutely ill patient, as well as the human experience of illness and normal growth and development—and much more. Increasingly called on to perform highly skilled technical-scientific and relational work, nurses must draw on nursing science and the natural physical and biological sciences as well as the social sciences and humanities.

Moreover, nurses learn and work under less-than-optimal circumstances. Nurses and nursing students must function within the complicated (and, many would say, chaotic and dysfunctional) environment of the U.S. health care system. Current health care institutions are not well designed for either good nursing and medical practice or education. For example, care of a critically ill patient in a hospital—a setting that is likely to be rapid-paced—typically involves layers of sophisticated technical supports and complicated titrations of multiple medications, all requiring the nurse's judicious monitoring and management. Further, disparities of health outcomes exist between the insured and the underinsured, of whom a disproportionate number are of lower economic means or belong to populations who encounter racism and other forms of cultural bias. With health care disparities at crisis proportions (Chao, Anderson, & Hernandez, 2009; Smedley, Stith, & Nelson, 2003), nurses struggle to uphold and transmit their core professional values of keeping patients safe and ameliorating human suffering. Because nurses are, as one student nurse in this study observed, the patient's "last line of defense" in a complex health care system, they must deploy a complex array of skills and knowledge, and do so with deep commitment to each patient's best interests.

A Crisis of Numbers

Since 1998, there has been a growing shortage of nurses (Buerhaus et al., 2007b; Buerhaus, Donelan, Ulrich, Norman, & Dittus, 2006). Moreover, during the mid-to-late 1990s, the number of students accepted to nursing schools dropped for five straight years, creating the conditions for a severe nursing workforce shortage that is predicted to grow in the coming decades as aging nurses, who make up the most populous demographic of the nursing workforce, retire: 45 percent are age fifty or older (Buerhaus et al., 2006). A 2007 survey reported that the hospital vacancy rate for registered nurses was 8.1 percent (American Hospital Association [AHA], 2007). The Bureau of Labor Statistics (Dohm & Shniper, 2007) projects a 23 percent increase in available nursing jobs by 2016, the largest increase for any occupation. Other projections show a similar increase in demand for nurses, from about two million full-time equivalents in 2000 to about 2.8 million in 2020, with a shortage of one million nurses to meet that demand (Health Resources and Services Administration/Bureau of Health Professions [HRSA/BHP], 2007).

To meet current and projected shortages, U.S. nursing education programs need to increase their capacity by approximately 90 percent (HRSA/BHP, 2006). However, nursing education programs, faced with a severe shortage of faculty, are hard pressed to expand; there is a dearth of baccalaureate-level nurses eligible to enter graduate programs to become nursing faculty. Even if prospective students could gain access to nursing schools and efforts to recruit foreign-trained nurses were successful, the shortage of nurses by 2020 would be about 340,000 (Auerbach, Buerhaus, & Staiger, 2007).

The implications of the shortage are profound. Nurses, the largest of the health care professional groups, spend the most direct time with patients; their role in health outcomes is therefore critical. Many studies agree that a shortage of qualified nurses decreases the quality of health care delivery (Aiken, Clarke, Sloane, Sochalski, & Silber, 2002; Aiken, Clarke, and Sloane, 2002; Cheung & Aiken, 2006). Ninety-three percent of hospital-based registered nurses report lack of sufficient staff and time to maintain patient safety, detect complications early, and collaborate with other health care team members (Buerhaus, Donelan, Ulrich, DesRoches, et al., 2007a; Buerhaus, Donelan, Ulrich, DesRoches, et al. 2007b). More nurses at the bedside could save thousands of patients' lives each year; a study published in the *Journal of the American Medical Association*, for example, reports that patients in hospitals having the highest patient-to-nurse ratios face up to 31 percent greater risk of dying (Aiken et al., 2002).

Improving Patient Care Outcomes Through Nursing Education

The numbers are indeed staggering. Yet they do not fully represent the urgent challenge to nursing and nursing education. More nurses alone, however, are not sufficient for improving patient care outcomes. Studies of nursing practice have demonstrated that better patient outcomes are achieved in hospitals staffed by a greater proportion of nurses with a baccalaureate degree and a smaller proportion of those with an associate degree (Estabrooks, Midodzi, Cummings, Ricker, & Giovannetti, 2005). Although currently 60 percent of nursing graduates hold the associate degree in nursing (ADN) as their highest degree, administrative nurses call for better-educated nurses even as they are forced by resource constraints to hire and reward nurses with an associate degree only and build large staffs through lower-paid ancillary positions (Orsolini-Hain, 2008).

The American Association of Nurse Executives and Nursing Chief Officers (AONE) calls for a better-educated nursing workforce, with nurses entering the profession from the baccalaureate level, and a reframing of the curriculum that leads to the bachelor of science in nursing (BSN). AONE's 2006 "Position Statement on Nursing Education" recommends: "The educational preparation of the nurse of the future should be at the baccalaureate level. This educational preparation will prepare the nurse of the future to function as an equal partner, collaborator and manager of the complex patient care journey. Given that the role in the future will be different, it is assumed that the baccalaureate curriculum will be re-framed" (American Organization of Nurse Executives [AONE], 2005).

Indeed, a major finding of our study is that a significant gap exists between today's nursing practice and the education for that practice, despite some considerable strengths in nursing education. Simply requiring more education will not be sufficient; the quality of nursing education must be uniformly higher. It is tempting to allow the current crisis related to a shortage of nurses to distract attention from the urgent need for increasing the quality and level of nursing science, natural and social sciences, and humanities currently offered in prelicensure programs. Even if there were no nursing shortage or nursing faculty shortage, nursing education would still need to change dramatically to meet the demands of current nursing practice.

In the course of our study, we found that the import of Johnson's findings (1988) about the quality of nursing education has only increased. Johnson noted significant differences in such areas as problem solving for nurses who have earned an associate degree or diploma compared to those with a baccalaureate degree. The need for better nursing education in science, humanities, social sciences, problem solving, teaching, and interpersonal capacities is, ten years later, even more acute. The rapidly developing field of practice demands preparation in more depth than is currently offered. The practice-education gap, already untenable, will continuously widen unless nursing education overhauls its approach to nursing science, natural and social sciences, and humanities. To be safe and effective practitioners nurses need to enter practice ready to draw on knowledge from a wide range of fields. Because practice will only become more complex over time, nurses must leave their formal programs prepared to be lifelong students, with the disposition and skills to be reflective practitioners and expert learners.

In prior studies of nursing education, researchers worried about the education-practice gap, that is, the ability of practice settings to adopt and reflect what was being taught in academic institutions. Now the tables are turned: nurse administrators and this research team worry about the practice-education gap, as it becomes harder and harder for nursing education to keep pace with rapid changes in a practice driven by research and new technologies (AONE, 2005). Although moving to baccalaureate-level education is a necessary first step, it will not be a sufficient catalyst for change unless baccalaureate nursing education programs are improved. Otherwise, the practice-education gap cannot be closed.

Opportunity at a Time of Crisis

The nursing shortage and the complex demands of practice put nursing education in a position of opportunity and responsibility to both expand and improve. Yet the pool of qualified faculty is too small and rapidly shrinking. Over the last decade, the number of available nursing faculty has decreased to the extent that schools face severe shortages of teachers. Faculty report that they simply cannot take on more students, even as schools are enlarging classes and scrambling to find more clinical sites, preceptors, and staff nurses who are willing to teach students. The American Association of Colleges of Nursing reported that 42,866 qualified applicants were turned away from baccalaureate schools of nursing in 2006 primarily because of a shortage of nursing faculty, clinical placement sites, and classroom space (American Association of Colleges of Nursing [AACN], 2007a). Similarly the National League for Nursing reported that in 2005, all schools of nursing rejected more than 147,000 qualified applications because of shortages of faculty, classroom space, and clinical placement for students (National League for Nursing [NLN], 2006). The number of applicants denied admission to nursing schools has increased sixfold since 2002 because of the faculty shortage (PricewaterhouseCoopers' Health Research Institute [PCHRI], 2007).

This is only the beginning of a precipitous drop in available faculty over the coming decade. Currently almost a third of all nursing faculty are over the age of fifty-five, and those with a doctoral degree are slightly older (U.S. Department of Health and Human Services [USDHHS], 2004). Among those under fifty-five, fewer have a doctorate, the preferred credential for teaching, and almost 50 percent of them are between the ages of forty-five and fifty-four (Berlin & Sechrist, 2002).

As faculty retire, nursing schools are losing some of their most experienced teachers and face the challenge of finding and mentoring new faculty. First, it will be a challenge to retain these new teachers; in most parts of the country, they can earn higher salaries in practice. Second, although those new to teaching often bring enthusiasm and up-to-date clinical knowledge, few graduating with a master's or doctoral degree have had any preparation for teaching. Faculty and administrators of graduate nursing programs have focused most of their attention for the past thirty years on developing nursing research. Graduate programs stopped making an effort to prepare future faculty for teaching and ignored the need to prepare new faculty to address the specific educational demands of teaching the complex practice of nursing. Few nursing faculty engage in the scholarship of teaching and learning, where faculty integrate their scholarship and teaching with research on teaching and learning (Boyer, 1990; Hatch, 2005; Huber & Hutchings, 2005). Nor are sufficient research dollars available to study nursing education. Yet, as our study confirmed, nursing education needs teachers with a deep nursing knowledge who also know how to teach and conduct research on nursing education. In this, nursing is not alone; lack of attention to preparing future faculty is endemic to graduate programs across the disciplines and professions (Walker, Golde, Jones, Bueschel, & Hutchings, 2008).

Nursing education's opportunity and responsibility extends to the curriculum and pedagogy, particularly in integrating clinical and classroom learning. As the burden of teaching increasingly falls on the shoulders of current nursing faculty, nurse leaders must support and revitalize faculty to teach better. If students experience high-quality teaching in nursing, more are likely to enter nursing education and be better teachers.

Hope for New Resources Uncertain

The faculty shortage poses serious challenges for schools, current students, and those thinking about entering nursing school. Moreover, at a time when a significant infusion of federal funds could help nursing education make some important steps forward, federal funding for programs is unreliable at best, and probably unlikely. In the more than forty years since the Nurse Training Act of 1964, funding for Title VII programs for health professions and Title VIII nursing workforce development programs has fluctuated. From 2001 to 2005, funds for Title VIII doubled to $150.67 million. In 2006, it was cut slightly, by 0.7 percent, to $149.68 million (AACN, 2008). However, the proposed 2009 federal budget projected 30 percent cuts to Title VIII funds (AACN, 2007b), and by late 2008 the federal government had pressing demands from and commitments to other sectors. This book goes to press at a time of economic crisis in the United States, and plans for changes in health care financing and delivery once again are at the forefront of the political debate and presidential agenda. Clearly, nursing leaders need to seize the opportunities for nursing education's potential contribution to health care reform inherent in the current economic and health care crises.

Lack of funds for nursing education presents one challenge. The public's vague and out-of-date understanding of what nurses must know and be able to do presents another. The knowledge, clinical judgment, and relational care that nursing demands are not readily visible. The trust that patients and the public put in nurses and nursing as a profession (Saad, 2006; American Nurses Association [ANA] Gallup Poll, 2008) may be well placed, but that trust is often based on an outdated, sentimental image of a relatively undereducated but nurturing and compassionate helper at the bedside. The fact that the profession is largely female may contribute to the persistent perception, in some quarters, of nurses as relatively unskilled but compassionate caregivers. Women still make up 94 percent of the profession (HRSA/BHP, 2006). The percentage of men enrolled in BSN programs, however, has risen only from 8.3 percent in 2003 to 9 percent in 2004 (AACN, 2007a). Unfortunately, the public, including legislators and other policy makers, underestimate the preparation necessary for today's nurses.

Toward a New Vision for Nursing Education

Even if nursing and nursing education were to receive an immediate influx of appropriately designated resources to address the shortages, along with appropriate policy changes, it would take many years to yield results. Thus, despite the enormous external challenges facing nursing and nursing education, we believe that change in nursing education must come now, from within the schools and programs and from within the profession. As nursing education copes with the pressures of these urgent shortages, the risk is to lower standards and aspirations. Indeed, at such a time of crisis it is especially critical to have a clear vision of what high-quality nursing education is and what programs must do to meet those standards, even when exigencies create pressure to move in the other direction. Outside assistance will not help if it focuses on expedience or is not intelligently guided.

We say this in the belief that too single-minded a focus on the crises of nurse and faculty shortages could lead nursing education in a direction opposite of what it most needs and away from its greatest strengths. Without addressing issues of the quality of nursing education, correcting the structural inadequacies will still not solve the problem. Indeed, well-meaning, large-scale efforts to increase student numbers, for example, could have as an unintended consequence weakening entry requirements and diluting local resources, such as clinical placements. Pressure to address the ever-burgeoning information of nursing science, bioethics, physiology, and other classroom subjects has already contributed to widespread reliance on, as one educator called it, "canned PowerPoint teaching." We believe that focusing on nursing education's potential to offer uniformly high-quality teaching and learning will revitalize current nurse educators and better prepare students to become the next generation of nurse educators.

To that end, for schools and the profession we offer a vision of transformation for nursing education that addresses the advanced knowledge, judgment, skills, and ethical standards needed by those who aspire to be nurses. Our major goal is to focus on changes in teaching and learning that will unburden overloaded curricula. On the basis of our examination of nursing education, we recommend approaches to teaching and student learning that will best prepare both today's and tomorrow's nurses. Indeed, we call for radical changes in nursing education, a radical new understanding of the nature of the curriculum and pedagogy (Sullivan & Rosin, 2008), and radical changes in the pathways to nursing licensure.

We offer this vision of nursing education transformed as the centennial anniversary of the publication of the highly influential "Flexner Report" approaches. That report, developed under the auspices of the Carnegie Foundation for the Advancement of Teaching in 1910, transformed medical education by bringing to it an expectation of scientific rigor and teaching based in academic settings. Other professions followed suit.

In 1997, the Carnegie Foundation conceived of the Preparation for the Professions Program to investigate once again how professionals are prepared to practice. Over the next ten years, national studies of the education of clergy, lawyers, engineers, nurses, and physicians were guided by then president Lee Shulman, and led by senior scholars William Sullivan and Anne Colby. Along with considerations of professional education, reports on educating clergy, lawyers, and engineers have already been published (Foster, Dahill, Golemon, & Tolentino, 2005; Sheppard, Macatangay, Colby, Sullivan, & Shulman, 2008; Sullivan, 2004; Sullivan, Colby, Wegner, Bond, & Shulman, 2007; Sullivan & Rosin, 2008). This national nursing education study, the national medical education study (Cooke, Irby, & O'Brien, forthcoming), and a comprehensive commentary on the program's findings will complete the series.

In *Work and Integrity*, the first report from the program, Sullivan argues that the professions are impoverished today because of the rise of a "technical professionalism" that has lost its traditional ethical commitment to the broader public good (Sullivan, 2004). Economic pressures and technology have altered the relationship between professionals and their clients and diminished the civic aspects of professional responsibility, as Sullivan observes:

> [A] democratic society ... draws heavily on the skills and moral sources of the professions. Particularly within a society like ours, in which the pull of utility and instrumental thinking—as in today's ascendant *business model* for institutions—is so strong, the professions are vital reminders that human welfare ultimately depends upon cultivation of values such as care and responsibility, which cannot be produced by self-interest alone. By focusing on the quality of their craft and the inventiveness of their practice, professionals provide an alternative model of what work can be: a contribution to public value, as well as a source of motivation and deep personal satisfaction [Benner and Sullivan, 2005, p. 78].

We believe that the enormous pressures on today's nursing profession—the chaotic U.S. health care system and the economic forces that drive it, shortage in the ranks of nurses, shortage of nursing educators, multiple pathways to the profession that discourage rather than encourage practicing nurses to complete postlicensure degrees—threaten to compromise nurses' ability to practice state-of-the-art nursing and enact the profession's core values of care and responsibility. As Sullivan explains: "Nursing and medicine have enjoyed positions of honor based on their social contract with the public that they serve. In exchange for bearing social responsibility for safe conduct with those who rely on their services, nurses and physicians, and indeed all professionals within the bounds of their legal regulations, have authority to control who enters their profession, how they are educated, and key aspects of how they conduct their work" (p. 80).

We share Sullivan's understanding of the social contract and the responsibility for those who enter the profession. It is thus imperative, we believe, to understand the education of those who aspire to be nurses and determine what interventions might counterbalance the prevailing forces. Accordingly, we framed our study of U.S. nursing education to examine how students are prepared as professionals in order to enter and uphold the social contract.

The Research Behind This Book

Using the same approach as the other Carnegie Foundation studies of professional education, the team studying nursing education reviewed the literature, conducted national surveys, and made direct observations of classroom and clinical teaching (see the Appendix for a description of the study methods).

In this study, we focused on the programs that prepare registered nurses (RNs). The research team conducted a series of three-day site visits at Riverside School of Nursing; Roberts Wesleyan College; Saddleback Community College; Samuel Merritt College; University of California, San Francisco; University of North Carolina at Chapel Hill; University of South Dakota; University of Washington; and Villanova University. As the list suggests, in spending time at these nine institutions, the team visited a variety of prelicensure programs, including those that grant the diploma, the associate degree, and the baccalaureate degree (both fast-track and traditional programs), as well as master's entry programs. Prior to the site visits, the team conducted extensive telephone interviews with administrators and faculty. On site, the team observed classes and interviewed administrators, faculty, staff, and students.

To deepen its understanding of teaching and student learning, the team asked each school to identify two courses, one introductory and one advanced, that it considered pivotal to the students' education. The team observed classes in these courses, interviewed the faculty about the goals of these courses and the faculty members' ideas about teaching and learning nursing practice, and interviewed a sample of students from the courses. We also observed students in clinical settings and skills and simulation laboratories. Additionally, the team conducted extensive interviews with senior students about their experiences in nursing.

To complement the site visits, the research included three national surveys of faculty and students, conducted in collaboration with leading nursing organizations: the American Association of Colleges of Nursing (AACN), the National League for Nursing (NLN), and the National Student Nurses' Association (NSNA). We have incorporated the findings from these surveys into this report, along with student and faculty comments. (See the survey instruments at www.CarnegieFoundation.org/nursingstudysurveys.)

The demands of practice are such that the professional must learn constantly and integrate knowledge, skilled know-how, and ethical comportment. Accordingly, during the site visits and in the surveys the research team asked about the relationship among these three apprenticeships. As the five Carnegie studies of education for the professions have consistently revealed, although the student's educational experience might focus on each apprenticeship separately or might emphasize one over the others, integrated learning and development across all three is necessary. An educational experience that carefully integrates these three apprenticeships, however, better prepares students to integrate them into professional practice, to use knowledge (Eraut, 1994) and skills appropriately in the context of commitment to values of care and responsibility. Throughout the book, we focus on the importance of integrating knowledge, skilled know-how, and ethical comportment during the educational experience.

Three Major Findings

Our site visits and surveys yielded a rich array of findings, both general and particular, about students' and educators' experience of nursing education and the extent of the practice-education gap. Among them are three major findings that have informed the focus of this book and our recommendations.

1. *U.S. nursing programs are very effective in forming professional identity and ethical comportment.* We found that nursing education is very strong in the pedagogies—particularly situated coaching and experiential learning—that are effective in helping students develop a deep sense of professional identity, commitment to the values of the profession, and to act with ethical comportment.

Interestingly, we found a significant difference between what educators and students articulate as their *understanding of* ethical comportment and the actual teaching of it: often educators and students described "ethics" primarily in terms of learning the principles of bioethics, with a focus on dilemma or breakdown ethics. Yet in the process of teaching and learning in clinical situations, educators and students focused on everyday ethical comportment, on becoming good practitioners and continuously improving their practice, always with the patient in mind.

We found that educators and students alike are engaged with and committed to good nursing practice organized to further the good of the patient. Although we found little or no cynicism or skepticism about the possibility and importance of improving nursing practice, we found much concern on the part of both faculty and students about the organizational and economic pressures that impede excellent nursing practice. Nursing students cite substandard nursing practice in their clinical practica as a major ethical concern in nursing school. On graduation, they are concerned that work overload and nursing staff shortages will press them to cut corners.

We applaud the depth of student and educator engagement with everyday ethical comportment and suggest that nursing education build on this strength and the effective teaching strategies of this aspect of nursing education.

2. *Clinical practice assignments provide powerful learning experiences, especially in those programs where educators integrate clinical and classroom teaching.* One strength of U.S. nursing education is that students work directly with patients and the health care team. Moreover, as they progress through their programs, they are given ever-increasing responsibilities in clinical situations.

When describing how they learned to become a nurse or "think like a nurse," students invariably pointed to clinical situations. As one student explained:

> Our clinical instructors are out on the floor at all times. They question us on everything about the patient we have taken on for that day. We have to learn about the labs and about the pathophysiology of our patient's diagnoses and rationale for treatment. If we are having a hard time figuring things out, we are given resources to do some research; and if by the end of our clinical rotation we have not figured it out, our instructors make it into a learning experience for the group. They are also out on the floor looking for things that we can do to gain the experience in skills that we have learned in labs so that we can become more comfortable in performing those skills. They are available at all times for questioning, too.

Students learn better when they are "lucky enough," as one put it, to be in a program where educators make an attempt to integrate the classroom and the clinical, especially when the instructors point to or, even more effectively, ask the student to draw on something from the classroom during clinical, or something from clinical in the classroom. The corollary: where the clinical and classroom instruction are not integrated or coordinated, students report a fragmented experience. A fragmented experience leads students to superficial understanding and precludes their ability to make astute clinical judgments in underdetermined situations. The acute shortage of nurse educators, however, diminishes the possibility of nurse educators who teach in both classroom and clinical settings. The shortage of staff nurses limits the supply of well-prepared clinical instructors to teach students in clinical settings.

3. *U.S. nursing programs are not generally effective in teaching nursing science, natural sciences, social sciences, technology, and humanities.* Nursing demands depth and breadth in domains in which knowledge is increasing, seemingly exponentially. Classroom faculty, in particular, try to cover a vast amount of information, yet the "to-learn" list lengthens as each new research finding is reported. As Tanner and others have noted, the nursing curriculum is additive (Tanner, 2004; Ironside, 2004); rather

than rework the material to reflect current practice, the faculty simply incorporates more.

Educators in nursing need to improve the teaching of nursing science, natural and social sciences, leadership, and humanities to ensure that all graduates are safe and effective clinicians, as well as lifelong learners who develop clinical knowledge (Porter-O'Grady & Malloch, 2003, 2007).

Nursing education uses the term *theory* to refer to this range of substantive knowledge about nursing care, nursing theories, nursing science, biology, chemistry, and physics as well as medical interventions that nurses need to master. The teaching we observed in "theory" classrooms was a sharp contrast to the skillful and effective pedagogical approaches we observed in clinical situations. The material is usually approached in a highly abstract way, with standardized lectures delivered mainly through slide presentations. Typically, the students are presented information about physiology, disease categories, signs, symptoms, interventions, and outcomes as taxonomies to be memorized—a pedagogical strategy that does not engage the student in imagining how such classification systems can be used in actual patient care.

We use "presented information" quite deliberately: in our observations and our conversations with students and faculty, we discovered widespread reliance on slide presentations and standardized lectures. In our site visits, we saw many classes begin with students opening their notebooks to an outline of the lecture and ending with the teacher at the front of the room having shown the last of dozens of slides. As the teacher glided from slide to slide, the students made notes in the margins of their course outlines, collectively turning their pages at every sixth slide. Discussion was cursory and some faculty even limited questions, not wanting to be pulled too far from the slide presentation.

Although this approach to teaching might seem an efficient strategy for staff-strapped programs and a tempting way to try to compress an ever-burgeoning body of information into a deliverable package, it is at cross-purposes with the way most adults learn, the way clinicians use knowledge as they think and act in ever-changing situations, and the way they will need to continue to learn as practitioners. Nursing, like all practice disciplines, relies on situated cognition and action. For example, on confronting a patient in acute respiratory distress, with low blood pressure and an extremely slow pulse, the nurse must take quick, definitive action and perform therapeutic interventions—based on deep understanding of the functioning of the lungs, the direction of the circulatory system, causes for slow heart rate, low blood pressure, and so on. In urgent situations demanding definitive quick response, the nurse needs to draw on knowledge, not abstract categories of clinical information, in order to act according to the needs of the patient and the best evidence for practice.

More troubling, we found a tenacious assumption that the student learns abstract information and then *applies* that information in practice. Developing knowledge that is to be *used* in a complex, high-stakes practice, such as nursing, calls for an ongoing dialogue between information and practice, between the particular and the general, so that students build an evidence base for care and thus learn to make decisions about appropriate interventions for the particular patient. The students must build a knowledge base at the same time they are developing a sense of salience—recognizing quickly what is most urgent, most important in each particular clinical situation.

Students do not fail to notice the sharp divide between the pedagogies of the classroom and the effective pedagogies of situated teaching in the clinical setting, and they find this divide perplexing not only because they learn so well in one arena and struggle to learn in another, but because the classroom experience is at odds with the strong ethos that results in deep commitment to professional values (and, as many students noted, deep personal transformation). Classroom teachers must step out from behind the screen full of slides and engage students in clinic-like learning experiences that ask them to learn to use knowledge and practice thinking in changing situations, always for the good of the patient.

The Plan of the Book: Paradigm Cases

The *strong instance* or paradigm case (Benner, 1994) illustrates a recognizable practice pattern. To illustrate how nursing education might build on its strengths and address its weaknesses in preparing students for professional practice, we structured this book around three paradigm cases of excellent teaching. We explore the habits, intents, and styles of instruction of three teachers* who have made key shifts in thinking about teaching and learning that led them to innovative and effective ways of teaching in the classroom. Although we observed and learned from many teachers

---

*We received written permission to reveal the names of the three paradigm case teachers: Lisa Day, Dianne Pestolesi, and Sarah Shannon. We were able to discuss our interpretations with these teachers and they agreed that our descriptions and understanding of their teaching adequately captured the aspects of their teaching presented in the book.

who extended our understanding of effective teaching and learning, these three nurse educators stood out because of their clear articulation of their teaching practice. They invite students to develop the sense of salience, clinical reasoning, and clinical imagination necessary to become effective and ethical nurses. Whether in the classroom or clinical setting, they strive to teach each student how to *be* a nurse who uses evidenced-based knowledge and cultivates habits of thinking for clinical judgment and skilled know-how. Their teaching is integrative and patient-centered. With a focus on formation, these teachers coach their students, engaging them in experiential learning to develop situated knowledge, skills, and ethical comportment. We augment the insights of these teachers with survey results, educator and student interviews, and examples from the many other classes we observed.

To put the paradigm cases in context, in Chapter One we describe in detail today's nursing practice and in Chapters Two and Three the current state of nursing education, focusing on what we learned about student experiences of clinical instruction and the classroom from our observations, interviews, and national surveys. To offer ways to address what we consider the most pressing issues of nursing education, we examine, in Chapter Four, the kind of teaching—and learning—that today's profession demands.

Most nursing practice requires a flexible and nuanced ability to interpret a not-yet-defined situation as an instance of something *salient* that should call forth an appropriate practitioner response. How does the student nurse learn to recognize possible good and less-than-optimal ends in actual clinical situations? In Part Two, we use a paradigm case to explore how the teacher helps students develop a sense of salience in clinical settings and how the teacher might then guide the students to draw on relevant research and consider possible interventions for the particular situation.

Good clinical judgment can never be reduced to the technical aspects of the situation or to a list of tasks to be accomplished. A nurse must consider, for example, the concerns of the patient and family as well as changes in the patient's clinical condition over time. In Part Three, we explore teaching to develop students' clinical imagination. Our paradigm case illustrates how student nurses might learn in an integrated fashion the medical and nursing implications of a situation—the pathophysiology of patients' clinical presentation and disease; diagnoses; medical therapies; the patients' experience; and physical, social, and spiritual recovery resources.

In Part Four, we describe teaching for professional formation and ethical comportment. We look in particular at how nurse educators support students in developing the vision, notions of good, and skilled use of the nurse's capacities that inform everyday care of patients.

As we explore each of these dimensions of nursing education, we consider particular aspects of nursing education that are in need of critique and revision, offering suggestions and examples drawn from our observations and interviews, the literature, other professions, and the learning sciences. In Parts One through Four, we offer specific recommendations for improvement at the program level. We close the book, in Part Five, with a set of recommendations for policy change that would not only support improved teaching and learning but better serve the profession. These recommendations will require the entire profession to work together to transform nursing education.

A Call to Action

Redesigning nursing education is an urgent societal agenda. Profound changes in nursing practice call for equally profound changes in education of nurses and preparation of nurses to teach nursing. The current climate rewards short-term focus, efficiency, and cost-savings that can compromise the quality of nursing education and patient care. The challenge will be to create health care institutions and management systems that educate nurses in a climate fostering professional attentiveness, responsibility, and excellence, where students learn that they have the authority, not just the responsibility, to practice.

To this end, we offer *Educating Nurses* as a starting place, a catalyst for conversation and debate, self-assessment, and above all change. Students, nurses, nurse educators, administrators of nursing schools, colleges and university leaders, administrators in health care settings, accrediting agency staff and leaders, and other leaders in the profession and education: our hope is that you find here a useful articulation of the problems and an inspiring vision for the future.

PART ONE

TRANSFORMATION, CRISIS, AND OPPORTUNITY

AT A TIME when nurses face new demands on their knowledge and responsibilities, the U.S. health care system is anticipating both a staggering shortage of nurses and a drop in the number of available faculty to educate new nurses. How, at this moment, can nursing education maximize its capacity and meet the needs of a transforming profession? How can teaching—and hence student learning—more effectively prepare students to enter a complex practice?

In the first of the four chapters in this part, we look at today's nursing practice in the United States. We consider the tremendous change the profession has undergone in recent decades and the challenge that nurses and nurse educators cite as their most pressing and constant concern: keeping up with the knowledge and skills that their work demands. We describe our findings in light of this challenge and others that nurse educators face, including the unintegrated structures of U.S. nursing education, faculty shortage, work overload, low faculty salaries, and limited clinical placements. We then turn, in Chapters Two and Three, to specific findings from our study about the experience of teaching and learning in clinical settings and the classroom.

We close Part One with a recommendation for a new approach to nursing education, one that builds on the considerable strengths we found and emphasizes teaching for a complex practice.

I

A PROFESSION TRANSFORMED

WE EMBARKED ON this study aware of the sweeping social and technological changes that have altered the context and substance of nurses' work since Lysaught's 1970 national study of nursing education. As professionals with expanding responsibilities in an increasingly complex field, even seasoned expert nurses must continuously learn across domains of knowledge and skill (Benner, Tanner, & Chesla, 2009; Porter-O'Grady & Malloch, 2003, 2007). This is an ethical mandate of the profession, a fact of professional life. An introduction to general science concepts is no longer adequate for understanding—and responding to—the complex health, illness, and treatment phenomena that nurses encounter in practice.

Nurses and nurse educators alike acknowledge the enormous pressure of expanded expectations for today's nursing practice. Continuing education for nurses is now mandated for relicensure, and state boards of nursing are giving attention to improving assessment of competency for continued licensure by state boards of nursing. At this point, nurses are left to their own self-assessment and selection of continuing education from a range of continuing education classes. Although most health care organizations have become centers of teaching and learning in their own right, they focus mainly on teaching new technologies and new regulations, both of which are necessary but do not offer the clinical knowledge and skilled know-how needed for a self-improving practice. Like staff nurses, nurse educators struggle to find continued education to keep up their clinical skills and ongoing faculty development for upgrading their pedagogical and curricular skills.

A Health Care System Transformed

Increasingly, the U.S. health care system has been concerned with profits, costs, and competition; health care is viewed as a commodity and even acutely ill patients are referred to as clients, customers, or even "product lines." Hospital-based care has changed dramatically, and care for the less acutely ill has shifted to the home and community. Reimbursement strategies are shifting from volume-based to "pay-for-performance" systems, and these systems depend on nurses to ensure that hospitals meet certain measures for quality, efficiency, and patient satisfaction (Lutz & Root, 2007), thereby positioning nurses as revenue sources rather than just part of hospital cost overhead.

Since the Lysaught Report was published, employment-based health care insurance has eroded and now only partially compensates highly technical care by public insurance programs. This change causes grave inequities in U.S. health care. At this writing, according to the U.S. Census Bureau's Current Population Survey, forty-seven million people in the United States are without health insurance. As it stands now, such an unwieldy system presents few incentives for preventive care for the uninsured, though for the past ten years managed care has sought to address prevention for insured patient populations (Institute of Medicine [IOM], 2008). Medical care itself tends to focus on acute episodic care because that is what most medical education programs emphasize. Moreover, U.S. society is ethnically and linguistically diverse, which increases the challenge of communication and understanding on the part of both health care workers and patients and their families. Another challenge is an aging population, and hospital patients reflect this fact, evidenced by recent increases in Medicare's Case Mix Index for inpatients (Lutz & Root, 2007), creating strain on care demands and economic resources of hospitals.

The revolution in information technology, the mushrooming of medical and nursing literature and technologies for accessing it, and the press to adopt electronic medical records while also protecting patient privacy have also changed the landscape of nurses' work. As sharing of expertise is facilitated by technology, care is now delivered by phone, computer, and across state lines and other geographic boundaries; further development along these lines will most certainly continue. Moreover, hospitals now care primarily for highly physiologically unstable patients and those whose ongoing therapies require careful monitoring, and often immediate adjustment of medications and therapies on the basis of the patient's responses to those therapies. As Marilyn Chow, vice president of patient care services at Kaiser Permanente, describes it, today's medical-surgical patient is the ICU patient of the 1970s (Robert Wood Johnson Foundation [RWJF], 2007). Today's nurses must work effectively in highly technical arenas within complex health care delivery systems, managing and titrating all the major medical therapies delivered in the acute care hospital, as well as in ambulatory care facilities and the home.

New Responsibilities

A tremendous shift of responsibility from physicians to nurses in all health care settings has occurred over the past sixty years. Physicians in many specialties now function primarily as diagnosticians and prescribers of treatment regimes. Nurses, patients, and family members administer these treatment regimens, usually under distant medical supervision. This requires a high degree of skill and knowledge. For example, to prepare medications nurses must understand multiple techniques of drug reconstitution, along with complex rules for drug compatibilities and incompatibilities. On the basis of the patient's response, the nurse must also adjust and titrate most therapies. Nurses are expected to perform complex, precise, and diverse technological interventions, keeping track of many machines and other devices. We noted in the staff break room of one pediatric unit that there are twenty intravenous (IV) infusion sets for children, all with distinct uses, many of which cannot be used interchangeably.

Given the nature of the interventions, the nurse's astute and early identification of changes in patients' physical condition in acute and long-term care facilities is critical to the safety and well-being of patients. The requirements of attentiveness and good clinical judgment multiply with the increasing acuity levels of hospitalized patients and with the many and diverse chronic illnesses now common in a rapidly aging population.

At the same time that this increase in the needs of hospitalized patients has come about, there has been a decline in the percentage of registered nurses (RNs) working in hospitals. The proportion of the nurse workforce employed in hospitals peaked in 1984 at 68.1 percent and has declined steadily to its current low of 56.2 percent employed registered nurses (HRSA/BHP, 2006), with more nursing care delivered in ambulatory care settings, the community, and in the home.

New Challenges

Despite these significant changes in the nature of health care work, including the need for physician nurse collaborations, health care settings remain hierarchical (Freidson, 1970), making communication across disciplines and the design of safe health care systems more complex. However, as "doctor's orders" change from specific directions to guidelines and parameters for nurses to judiciously adjust therapies according to the patient's responses, clear communication and coordination between nursing and medicine becomes imperative. Studies have shown improved patient outcomes when the communication channels between nurses and physicians work well (Carroll, 2007; Arford, 2005; Baggs et al., 1999; Baggs, 1989), and a number of studies have demonstrated that poor nurse-physician communication is linked to medication errors (Kohn, Corrigan, & Donaldson, 2000; Leape, 1994), patient injuries (Page, 2004), and patient deaths (Tammelleo, 2001, 2002).

At cross-purposes to this new need for clear and precise communication within an interprofessional health care team is education for the various members of the team. Nursing, medicine, physical therapy, and other health care professions educate their students in academic silos, isolated from one another and hence largely ignorant of the expertise of those with whom they will need to work closely and seamlessly. Julie Gerberding, former director of the Centers for Disease Control and Prevention, has called for changing how doctors, nurses, and other health care providers are educated: "I believe that what we really need in this country are schools of health. . . . If we are seriously thinking about building a health care system, then we need to be training professionals in a collegial and collaborative manner" (Fox, 2007). However, both the Carnegie Foundation's study of medical education and this study of nursing education found that even though there is agreement that more collaborative medical and nursing education is needed, this coordination is practically absent in curriculum plans, and informal collaboration is infrequent, even in clinical settings where nurses and doctors are both in training.

New Opportunities

Over the past two decades in particular, nursing has made important academic strides through growth in programs in nursing research housed in graduate nursing schools and the availability of federal funds to support the research programs. The National Center for Nursing Research was established in 1986 by the Health Research Extension Act of 1985 (Public Law 99–158; see Kjervrik, 2006), and in 1993 the center became a full-fledged institute within the National Institutes of Health (NIH), the National Institute of Nursing Research (NINR).

These developments fostered important increases in the quantity, and quality, of research done by nurses. Exciting research is shedding new light on such issues as the psychosocial aspects of coping with illness, patient education, and physiological and behavioral aspects of health promotion and chronic illness management. There is a growing body of nursing research on symptom management, end-of-life care, care of the aged and chronically ill, genomics, and more.

The NINR research agenda continues to be directed primarily toward basic and applied research related to patient care; promotion of health and prevention of illness; reducing health disparities; understanding individual, family, and community responses to acute and chronic illness and disability; and end-of-life care. Patient care research also addresses ethical and public policy concerns that affect delivery of patient care. This research sponsorship by NIH moved nursing education and research into a new era. The impact of research-intensive nursing schools on nursing science has been extensive, and these schools led a shift in the primary focus of nursing research from nursing education to patient care. The shift was much needed, but it went too far; researchers can no longer continue to focus on one at the expense of the other. Hence one purpose of this book is to revitalize research programs in nursing education and increase efforts and resources for better faculty preparation in graduate school and ongoing faculty development and research and development of nursing education.

Integrating Nursing Science and Caring Practices

In 1970, Lysaught complained of overemphasis on the expressive, emotional, nurturing side of nursing, which at the time was usually dismissed as a feminine trait instead of being understood as facets of deep knowledge and complex skills. Lysaught worried that underemphasis of the technical and instrumental work of nurses, exemplified by such therapies as the high-impact work of starting closed-chest resuscitation, or titration of potent intravenous medications, would lead to undervaluing of the knowledge and skill required for nursing practice.

Lysaught was concerned about nurses representing themselves and being understood as having exceptional relational skills, which obscured their scientific and technical capacities. He read caregiving practices as noninstrumental "niceties" that somehow did not really count as knowledge and skill at all compared to medicine's therapeutic and curative enterprise. He offered an oversimplified choice: nurses had to represent themselves either as highly effective interventionists who were knowledgeable and skillful in science and technology or as nonskilled nurturers—two mutually exclusive options, neither of which accurately represents the complexity of nursing care. A decade later, second-wave feminists in the 1980s sought to correct the marginalization of caring practices, arguing that caring practices and relational work, which foster growth, empowerment, and liberation, are indeed knowledge-based and complex (Benjamin, 1988; Benner & Wrubel, 1989; Ruddick, 1989; Whitbeck, 1983). This setting of instrumental, technical-scientific work in opposition to relational work is still perpetuated when nurses present their practice as primarily instrumental, or relational and nurturing work (Nelson, 2006). They ignore the fact that interpersonal relational and technical-scientific knowledge are intricately intertwined in nursing and medical instrumental work. Typically in professional fields, as the technical and instrumental nature of the knowledge and skilled know-how increase, so does the need for effective communication and relational skills.

Lysaught correctly read his current culture, but he could not predict how much technology and economics would change health care, the extent to which nurses' shift to high-stakes technical therapies also increased the need for higher levels of skill necessary to communicate with patients and families, and how crucial relational work would be for effective highly technical patient care (Benner, 1984; Benner, 2000; Benner, Tanner, & Chesla, 2009). He could not have anticipated the deep and complex education that nurses would need—the array of knowledge from the nursing sciences, natural sciences, social sciences, and humanities; skills of practice; and ethical comportment—to function as professionals. He did not confront the problem of splitting off the instrumental and the emotional skills in thinking or in any complex practice (Damasio, 1994).

This study considers the nature of nursing practice in ways that Lysaught perhaps could not recognize at the time he was writing. It joins the other Carnegie Preparation for the Professions studies to examine the deep and complex education that professionals need. All of these studies use the metaphor of "apprenticeship" to capture the experiential learning that requires interaction with a community of practice, situated coaching by teachers, and demonstration of aspects of a complex practice that are not easily translated. For example, a student cannot read about bundling premature infants as a procedure in a book and then be expected to bundle a premature infant without some professional guidance for how to avoid damaging the underdeveloped muscles of a fragile premature infant who is easily overstimulated and injured. In a professional practice, one does not easily translate what one learns from textbooks and research articles into skilled know-how and the ability to engage in clinical reasoning across changes over time. Nor is it easy to gain a sense of salience, which is when a practitioner can discern what is more or less important in a clinical situation.

To explain how students learn during their professional education, we suggest three broad and inclusive apprenticeships that refer to the whole domain of professional knowledge and practice: (1) an apprenticeship to learn nursing knowledge and science, (2) a practical apprenticeship to learn skilled know-how and clinical reasoning, and (3) an apprenticeship of ethical comportment and formation. We use the word *apprenticeship* with some caveats. They are "high-end" apprenticeships, and by this we do not mean slavish imitation of master teachers or coaches; instead creative and critical thinking, questioning, and innovation are central to learning a professional practice. Nor do we mean on-the-job training. We also do not mean apprenticing to one master teacher or institution. High-end apprenticeships should not be confused with Bloom's taxonomy (1968), which uses teaching concepts that involve cognitive, affective, and motor pathways to teach or learn a concept or skill at the daily level of teaching specific content. Bloom points to acquiring new skills or knowledge through sight, emotion, and action pathways as a central principle of learning anything new. Indeed we agree with his integrative point about using all perceptual pathways for more effective learning. Finally we acknowledge that the term *apprenticeship learning* is particularly controversial in nursing. We thought long and hard about the advantages and disadvantages of using it. Our use of the term is not a reference to the historical apprenticeship model of learning most common in diploma schools of nursing until the early 1970s, when nursing moved into the academy. In the older model of apprenticeship of hospital training programs, students furnished the major portion of care to patients and were seen not as engaged in a program of education. In the service-driven diploma programs of forty years ago, classroom instruction and planned, tutored clinical experiences were subordinated to hospital demands for an inexpensive, and relatively unskilled, labor pool to care for patients.

Even though we want to avoid the connotations of abuse, domination, and control often associated with apprenticeship learning, we still hold on to the notion of learning by doing, observing, and participating in a community of practice. Instead, by *apprenticeship* we mean a range of integrative learning required for any professional that includes (1) instantiating, articulating, and making visible and accessible key aspects of competent and expert performance; (2) giving learners a chance for supervised practice; (3) coaching in the supervised practice to help students understand, reflect on, and articulate their practice, particularly the nature of particular clinical situations; (4) helping novice students recognize the priorities and demands embedded in particular clinical situations so that they gain a sense of salience, that is, what must be attended to and addressed in relation to the significance and urgency in the particular clinical situation; and (5) reflection on practice to help the student develop a self-improving practice. Apprenticing oneself to a health care team, a community of practice, and even to patients and families is essential for learning to grasp the nature of the clinical situation, gaining situated understanding, skill, and the ability to *use* knowledge.

We draw heavily on Lave and Wenger (1991) in describing experiential learning, but we stop short of fully adopting their term "legitimate peripheral performance." It is almost impossible to limit learning nursing and medical practice to peripheral performance. Early in their clinical learning nursing and medical students must enter high-stakes learning situations and are called on to perform appropriately and knowledgeably in response to the immediate needs of their patients. Nurse educators deliberately engage students directly in practice as soon as possible, rather than have students just observe or shadow other nurses. Though their limited knowledge prevents central participation and agency in the beginning of their practice, they still engage in high-stakes learning situations where they must act responsibly and integrate the complex knowledge, skill, notions of good, and ethical comportment that nurses must learn to use in practice.

As the Carnegie studies have pointed out, professional schools are hybrid institutions; they are part of the tradition of "cognitive rationality" at which the academy excels, and they are part of the world of practice, where skilled know-how marks expert practitioners. Ideally, each of the three professional apprenticeships would be emphasized equally and taught integratively, as the learner changes from a layperson to professional nurse. However, the practicalities of presentation demand that we look at the three apprenticeships as distinct domains. Let us keep in mind, though, that once the three apprenticeships are separated, it is hard to get them back together again.

Acquiring and Using Knowledge and Science

Whether it is microbiology, interpretation of laboratory results, how culture and health practices intersect, or the influences of family and community on an individual's illness experience, nurses must acquire and use knowledge from many fields.

Patients in acute care, "the ICU patient of the 1970s," are extremely unstable, and nurses must be able to grasp the significance of subtle yet meaningful changes; a keen perception of subtle changes in patients, for example, contributes to astute, possibly life-saving actions. At the same time, to act appropriately nurses now need sophisticated understanding of chemistry, physiology, pathophysiology, microbiology, physics, genetics, and more. For example, nurses need to understand physics as it is relevant to patient care. It is no longer sufficient for nurses to be concerned with oxygen exchange within the lungs; they must know how oxygen and nutrients are being taken up and used at the cellular level. Along similar lines, nurses must use knowledge from biochemistry to thoroughly understand acid-base balance, electrolytes, and solutions, biochemical cascades, coagulation, and fibrinolysis. Similarly, wherever the site of practice, nurses need a solid knowledge of microbiology, such as human-pathogen interactions and evidence-based use of antibiotics in the context of a worldwide problem of antibiotic resistance and increasing numbers of patients who are immuno-compromised.

Today's nurses are expected to know more about interpretation of laboratory findings than simply the normal and abnormal ranges. To use current intravenous drugs, which must be carefully monitored and titrated, nurses need sophisticated knowledge of pharmacokinetics, hemodynamics, and cardiac function. For practice in all areas of the acute care hospital, nurses must be prepared to administer, monitor, and evaluate these therapies.

On the horizon lie increased use of genomic medicine and pharmacodynamics. To keep pace with the care implications of research on both genetic markers and gene therapies related to multiple gene diseases, nurses will need to understand basic, medically relevant genomics. There will be an increasing need for dedicated, well-educated genetic counselors as genomics becomes more prevalent in everyday health care; nurses will need to be prepared to convey the goals and risks of genetic therapies for patients with chronic illnesses. Other areas in human genomics will also be more important for nurses, as they will be expected to educate patients about genetics related to diseases and other conditions, from birth through later life.

In short nurses need to be able to draw on new knowledge from fields traditionally taught, such as pathophysiology, and from new fields, such as genomics.

Using Clinical Reasoning and Skilled Know-How

Nurses use knowledge from many fields to help them grasp the medical and nursing implications of a situation, "read" a patient's condition over time, manage time and resources, and master ever-changing, increasingly complex technical skills. They must also develop relational and communication skills for delivering patient care, educating patients, and being an effective health care team member. Nurses must be able to make a case to colleagues or other health professionals on behalf of a patient. Thus writing and speaking well are among the essential skills of nursing practice. Nurses need improved education in oral and written communication so that they can communicate effectively at several levels and in varied circumstances. Those in leadership positions, for example, must be particularly effective communicators, because they also create institutional directives and policy.

Nurses now perform extensive patient and family education and work with health care team members, so they must be able to articulate their practical clinical knowledge. Nurses must speak and write clearly about their narrative understanding of patient-family illness experiences and concerns. They must be able to draw out and understand "stories of illness," or patient illness narratives, as well as physical histories of injuries or disease. They must be able to make a clinical case for reporting changes in a patient's condition or concerns and in synthesizing patient and family information from many sources. The nurse's narrative understanding is also essential for the patient's experience of care; patients who feel known, whose stories inform the care they receive from nurses, experience better care than those who feel objectified and unknown.

Whether they are reading patients and a situation, talking to family members, or working with other members of the health care team, nurses need astute clinical judgment informed by attuned relational skills, such as listening, as well as reflecting and interpreting the patient's concerns and experience.

Ethical Comportment and Formation

Above all, nurses need a good grasp of everyday ethical comportment, demonstrating appropriate use of knowledge, skills of care and relations, and communication with patients and colleagues. They need to be as skilled at responding ethically to error as they are in making ethical decisions and solving problems. Nurses need the skill of ethical reflection to discern moral dilemmas and injustices created by inept or incompetent health care, by an inequitable health care delivery system, or by the competing claims of family members or other members of the health care team.

To this end, nurses must develop moral resources for nursing care and understand a range of ethical theories. Nurses cope with difficult ethical problems that might attract attention locally or even nationally as well as issues of "everyday ethics," such as confronting substandard care. They need ethical skills and commitment to face such large-scale ethical problems as the social impact on health of violence and pollution and socioeconomic, racial, or ethnic disparities in health care and health outcomes. Nurses also have an important role at the policy level, where they must face large-scale ethical dilemmas. For these they must bring similar skills and knowledge from their unique perspective to participate in their rightful place in the health care policy arena.

Integration of Knowledge, Skilled Know-How, and Ethical Comportment

As experts in high-stakes professional practice, nurses constantly integrate their knowledge and skills according to particular patient care concerns, demands, resources, and constraints. Thus reasoning through a particular patient's condition and situation is a core skill for nurses. Because patients' conditions can change rapidly, with life and death in the balance, nurses need to be able to grasp changes in the patient's condition and integrate their knowledge and skills quickly and confidently.

Thus, as we note at the outset of this discussion, today's practitioner must continuously be able to draw on all they learn in each of the professional apprenticeships (cognitive, skilled know-how, ethical comportment) and integrate them in practice. She must hold her knowledge and skills in a fluid or semipermeable way, drawing on them as the situation requires. She must also be able to articulate what leads her to decide on a particular action. For example, a nurse expert in detecting heart arrhythmias on a unit where all patients' cardiac functioning is monitored will notice only aberrations in sound patterns, while the familiar normal sounds remain in the background of attention. She must then be able to describe what she hears to others. Whereas in many skill situations experts do not need to articulate their perspectives before taking action, the nurse must often make a clinical case for interventions to health care team members, presenting solid evidence and interpreting the clinical situation in order to get coordinated, accurate, and timely action from the team. In emergencies when no physician is available, the nurse must be able to articulate clearly the reason for using a standing order or protocol, or going beyond the usual boundaries of nursing practice to save a patient's life or prevent harm. Acting judiciously and rapidly on behalf of the patient is expected and defensible when it is critical for the patient's survival. Recognizing the unexpected, when predictable expectations of patients' recovery are not met, is also a hallmark of expert practice (Benner et al., 2009).

At the heart of learning any practice discipline, whether it be clergy, medicine, law, engineering, or nursing, lies the need for situated cognition (Lave & Wenger, 1991), or the chance to think in particular clinical situations. Such a chance helps practitioners cope when they confront practice, where situations are ill defined and multifaceted, and each situation has many possibilities for understanding and action. The professional seeks an optimal grasp of the nature of the situation from which she can proceed in her assessments and discernment (Chan, 2005). Excellent practice requires interpretation and an imaginative grasp of the possibilities inherent in the particular situation, as well as appropriating relevant knowledge for the particular demands of the situation. For nurses, the capacities to see and to act require imaginative understanding and rapport with patients. In their formation, nurses encounter their own coping in the context of identifying others' ways of handling difficult life experiences such as suffering, dying, and emotional responses of patients, including anger, helplessness, and fear. Equally formative are students' newly developing capacities to recognize subtle signs, symptoms, and complex physiological reactions. This is why active learning and emphasis on formation are so central to professional nursing education. Student nurses need rich opportunities to continue to learn, develop their practice, and articulate it both as individual nurses and members of a health care team.

Nursing educators excel at teaching by example and with situated coaching in the clinical area, or the coaching of students in particular clinical situations. Currently students' integrative learning occurs mostly through situated coaching and from learning through the experience of practice, where students learn from other practitioners, patients, and their families. Thus we identify situated coaching as a signature pedagogy in nursing education.

Nevertheless, students experience a sharp separation of classroom and clinical teaching, and we suggest that nursing educators need to drop the current extreme divide between their teaching in classroom and clinical settings. Nursing students can, and should, develop ethical comportment in clinical and classroom settings, acquire skilled know-how and clinical reasoning in both, and build nursing knowledge in classroom and clinical settings, preferably integrated. With better integration, students learn that practice is a way of knowing in its own right. In other words, innovation and new questions flow bidirectionally, from theory and science to and from practice.

A System Inadequate to the Task

Given the enormous changes in and complexity of current nursing practice and practice settings, are nurses entering practice equipped with the knowledge and skills for today's practice and prepared to continue clinical learning for tomorrow's nursing? The answer to this question was the central goal of our study: We found that, in short, the answer is no.

Nursing practice works deliberately in the in-between social spaces of medical diagnosis and treatment and the patients' lived experience of illness or prevention of illness in their particular life, family, and community. In general, we found that nursing school curricula are weak in the natural sciences, technology, social sciences, and humanities. The curricula are weak in the experiences that enable students to work effectively with those of different cultures, races, socioeconomic status, religious affiliation, gender, or sexual preferences.

Rapid changes in science, technology, and clinical practice require a higher level of scholarship and more clinically oriented teaching in all arenas of nursing education. Like many academics, nurse educators focus on their students' acquisition of knowledge; however, nurses must know how to use that knowledge in practice (Eraut, 1994). Teaching strategies, such as situated cognition and thinking in action, are essential in classrooms, simulation laboratories, and clinical settings.

We also found that students were not well prepared to continue their clinical learning. The "pedagogies of inquiry" are weak in nursing schools. By this we mean strategies that help students learn to develop the habit and skills of following up on or working through clinical puzzles and concerns or issues that show up in clinical assignments. Pedagogies of inquiry also require learning research skills, and access to existing research databases (Malloch & O'Porter-Grady, 2006). We found serious gaps in students' knowledge about how to answer clinical questions using the literature or the resources they have at hand, such as use of information systems, databases, and asking for help from a colleague in another discipline. Thus the skills of inquiry that nurses have as they enter practice are weak, a situation which hampers their learning over the course of their careers.

Our surveys revealed that students and faculty alike think that nursing students are not adequately prepared for their first job. To be sure, schools cannot adequately prepare students for practice in all places; each practice site demands that nurses learn a significant amount of local, specific knowledge. For this, newly graduated nurses should have at least a one-year, high-quality, postgraduate residency in a specific practice setting. Yet postgraduate residencies alone will not suffice if the student lacks a strong basis in the scientific and humanities knowledge needed for today's practice. Moreover, as noted earlier in this chapter, students need to develop excellent inquiry and research skills because they will continue to learn new knowledge and develop their practice over the course of their career. Thus schools can never adequately prepare their graduates for the full range of complexity of practice, with its ongoing changes in technology and nursing knowledge. However, they can prepare students to enter practice ready to integrate knowledge, skilled know-how, and ethical comportment and to continue to engage in self-directed learning at a highly developed level.

The current system of nursing education is not adequate to prepare today's nurses for the immediate future. We found that many teachers and students are dissatisfied with the teaching preparation of current nursing faculty. Further, we note that current graduate nursing programs do not systematically offer opportunities for learning how to teach, such as classes or seminars on teaching or guided teaching assistantships. Educators reported that they do not have enough time or opportunities to reflect or discuss the scholarship of their teaching. The combination of lack of basic teacher preparation in graduate nursing schools and limited faculty development conspires to thwart the scholarship of teaching in nursing.

In 1990 Ernest Boyer and his colleagues at the Carnegie Foundation published *Scholarship Reconsidered*, which called for a "more inclusive view of what it means to be a scholar," one that included the scholarship of teaching, along with the more accepted types of scholarship of discovery, integration, and application (Boyer, 1990). Boyer's books and the subsequent work by the Carnegie Foundation scholar Mary Huber and the vice president of the foundation Pat Hutchings touched off new interest in what it means to take up teaching as scholarship and generated important questions about teaching and learning. The International Society for the Scholarship of Teaching and Learning, created as a response to Boyer's reports, calls for institutions to make time for faculty to pursue and recognize the scholarship of teaching and learning. The scholarship of teaching and learning includes developing new approaches to curricula; new, innovative, integrative or interdisciplinary courses; new teaching and learning delivery methods such as distance education; new instructional innovations such as simulation; and evaluation strategies to capture the processes of *using knowledge*. Other approaches to teaching and learning include more integrative pedagogies, development of curricula, and restructuring of the access to practice skills and knowledge to make teaching and learning more relevant to the work within a particular discipline.

We found that multiple educational pathways for entering nursing students exacerbate the problems we identify. It is important to note that our findings about the strengths and weaknesses of nursing education are not particular to any of the various program types or settings. However, as we shall discuss, the varied pathways create limitations on student learning and disincentives for students to pursue the BSN. In general, we found that although nursing is to be lauded for being accessible through its multiple points of access to education, the system of multiple pathways into the profession, each with its own requirements for student graduation, does not support the high-quality teaching and learning so crucial to nurses' preparation and improved patient outcomes.

Multiple Pathways

Perhaps no other issue in nursing education and practice is as contested as the multiple educational pathways into the profession, the diverse range of nursing programs that prepare students to sit for the licensure exam to become a professional nurse. In nursing, the first professional degree can be an undergraduate degree, but it does not have to be. Students may sit for the National Council Licensure Examination for Registered Nurses (NCLEX-RN) upon completion of an approved generic baccalaureate program (four years), or a fast-track second baccalaureate degree program (fourteen to eighteen months), or a master's program designed for students who already have a baccalaureate degree in another discipline (three years), or an associate degree program (a program that takes at least three years and usually more to complete), or a two-to-three-year diploma program offered through freestanding schools of nursing affiliated with and sponsored by hospitals or health care systems.

Unlike medical students, who have a relatively uniform experience—an undergraduate degree, a core of prerequisites that do not vary much from school to school, and a standardized premedical admissions examination—nursing students in these various pathways do not share equivalent, or even similar, prerequisite courses. Nor have they taken a common entrance examination. Some students are recent high school graduates and others graduated from high school—or even college—decades before they started nursing school. Unlike medical students, many nursing students pursue their studies part-time or full-time.

As we considered how to convey particular findings about students' experience of nursing education, with its multiple points of entry and pathways and varied curricula and timeframes, we found it unwieldy to make comparisons based on a student's place in a program, or year in school. Although the core nursing courses are generally designed to be completed in two years, the amount of time that elapses significantly depends on the student's program and whether she is attending full-time or part-time.

Historical Origins

Prior to 1960, nurses were educated almost exclusively in hospital-based diploma programs. In these service-driven programs, classroom instruction and planned, tutored clinical experiences—the basic components of today's nursing curriculum—were not only limited but also subordinate to the hospital's need for an inexpensive and relatively unskilled labor pool. The hospital nursing administrator directed the school and relied on students to work. Indeed, because students administered the major portion of care to patients, they were not seen so much as engaged in a program of education as supplying an extra pair of working hands.

In 1948, the year that Esther Lucille Brown published *Nursing for the Future*, there were a few schools that offered a baccalaureate in nursing. Brown argued that U.S. nursing education should occur in institutions of higher education. The first associate degree programs were created in 1958, and within twenty-five years the number of associate degree nursing programs grew from seven to nearly seven hundred (Mahaffey, 2002), coinciding with creation of the U.S. community college. Community colleges housed technical nursing programs, and most programs were publicly funded. The number of diploma schools, most of which were privately funded, declined precipitously (IOM, 1983). The Nurse Training Act of 1964 (Public Law 88–581) initiated an important stream of funding for nursing education. During the 1960s and 1970s, state and local funds increased, along with federal funds, for nurse education, teaching facilities, student loans, projects for strengthening nurse education programs, "formula payments," and training (IOM, 1983). By 1974, the number of nurses educated in a college or university equaled those educated in a diploma program.

The Rise of Community College Programs

Larger forces of economics and policy, the growth and trajectory of higher education in the United States, and the U.S. health care system all play out in nursing education. Limited funding for nursing education discourages students from entering and completing BSN programs and creates enormous pressure on community colleges (which are more affordable) to accommodate students pursuing the ADN. Moreover, students are eager to enter practice, and the current policy for licensure not only makes it possible for them to do so but also encourages them to enter the profession with the minimum credential, which they can earn through a community college.

Indeed, they have been doing so in greater numbers. In 2006, for the first time, the majority of the 23,278 graduates from nursing schools or programs who took the NCLEX-RN were the 13,444 graduates of associate degree programs, or about 60 percent of the total number. Community colleges now produce the largest number of practicing RNs (National Council of State Boards of Nursing [NCSBN], 2005).

Yet a critical shortage of nursing faculty limits the number of students these programs can serve. Although community college programs are intended to be two-year courses of study and are presented to the public as such, with a year of prerequisites and a long waiting list for entry into programs and classes, many students need three years or more to complete the degree. For example, community college students in our national survey reported spending on average nineteen to twenty-four months in ADN programs, exclusive of the time they might spend on school or program prerequisites; in another recent study, ADNs who entered practice without the BSN reported an average of 3.69 years in an ADN program (Orsolini-Hain, 2008). In some states, programs are so constrained by shortages of instructors that students may need as many as four to six years to earn the degree; courses are simply not available. Moreover, because their funding is based on student count alone community colleges usually lack funding to fully support the high costs of the nursing students' intensely supervised clinical training.

We note that the time and expense to earn the ADN alone discourages many students from continuing their studies and completing a baccalaureate degree, especially when they can readily get a relatively well-paying position as a staff nurse. As a result, only about 21 percent of ADNs go on for further formal education (Orsolini-Hain, 2008), often missing such important areas as pediatrics, community health, and more extensive attention to leadership, as well as courses in the humanities and health policy.

Nurse educators have relied too much on general research on education and have developed little domain-specific research on teaching nursing. Approaching nursing education through the lens of domain-specific teaching would suggest that different pedagogies are needed if students are to develop a deep understanding of nursing science, relevant natural and social sciences, and humanities to be used in nursing practice. To complement the effective clinical experience, students need to experience effective classroom pedagogies that allow them to imagine how they will respond in clinical situations. As we describe in Parts Two through Four, presenting unfolding case studies, narrative accounts of clinical experiences, or simulation of cliniclike situations would bring into the nursing school *classroom* the kinds of teaching strategies (such as coaching for situated cognition, action, and articulation) that are the signature pedagogies of clinical nursing education.

Making the classroom, skills, and simulation labs places for rich, experiential learning that encourages students to imaginatively and creatively use knowledge in particular situations offers opportunities for lasting learning that is more complex than any competency list or single theory (Taylor, 1985a). Nursing students need opportunities to safely practice reading situations, imaginatively see possibilities, and draw on knowledge in particular clinical situations.

It is extremely valuable for schools of nursing to link with the resources of schools of education, but such linkage does not solve the research problems of how best to teach for nursing practice. As guardians of the discipline and practice of nursing, nurse educators need to engage in research and development of nursing-specific pedagogies and curricular strategies (Golde & Walker, 2006).

Meeting the Demand for Nursing Education

The demand for entry into nursing school is felt throughout the system. As varied as the prerequisites for entry into a nursing program might be (which raises questions about what, exactly, the appropriate prerequisites are), we note that nursing schools are commonly oversubscribed, with a long waiting period for admission. More students are coming to nursing school (to diploma, community colleges, and BSN programs alike) with a baccalaureate or even an advanced degree from another discipline. The accelerated curricula that are designed to accommodate these students do not necessarily succeed; many students need science and social science prerequisites oriented to the nursing school curriculum.

Although a stated goal of the U.S. nursing profession (Sullivan, 2004) is diversity that more closely reflects the U.S. patient population, African American, Hispanic American, Asian American, and Native Americans make up only 9 percent of nurses, and men constitute only 6 percent of the profession. We found that nursing programs have recruitment for diversity as a goal, but the students and educators are predominantly female and Caucasian.

Raising a Bar Too Low for Entry Standards

Whether it is an indication of the continued pressures of a nursing short-age or a result of lack of appreciation for nurses' increasing responsibility, judgment, knowledge, work, and autonomy, it is puzzling to find low stan-dards for entry to nursing school. We found wide variation in prerequisites for nursing programs, and this raises a question about what coursework students need before they start the nursing portion of their education. To compound the problem, in many regions of the country prerequisite courses for nursing school are oversubscribed and require a long waiting period for admission.

Nursing Prerequisites

There is a pressing need to expand the number of available courses and reevaluate the prerequisites for nursing education. To address variation in quality and content, a national advisory group consisting of nursing fac-ulty, clinicians, physicians, pharmacists, and expert science teachers need to agree on content that prerequisite courses must cover before students can start a nursing program. This group would select and order the most clinically relevant science instruction for nursing and require a range of courses to give students a broad grounding in liberal arts (humanities, natural sciences, and social sciences). In addition, this group must agree on prerequisites for the many students who are coming to nursing school with a baccalaureate or advanced degree, many of whom have completed extensive coursework in natural sciences, social sciences, and humanities. We foresee that this advisory group would meet periodically to update the science course prerequisites.

Nursing also faces another significant challenge—as well as an opportunity—in the form of its multiple pathways. In the next section, we call for structural changes that would address this: requiring the BSN as the first step on a continuum of education, raising the standards for licensure.

The BSN and Beyond

Students who choose to pursue a BSN, whether through an accelerated program or a traditional one, have the advantage of learning more, and in greater depth. The general education courses that are part of the BSN curriculum expose students to further opportunities to learn to write clearly, marshal evidence for an argument, conduct research, make connections across various domains of knowledge, articulate issues of ethics, and continue to develop knowledge and skills independently.

Thus, as we advocate in the final section of this book, among the structural changes we believe nursing education must make is to streamline community college nursing programs and create a seamless and immediate articulation with baccalaureate programs so that they can meet the heavy demand for affordable entry into the nursing education system, while not forcing students to spend three to five years on an associate degree. We also recommend that students complete their ADN and their BSN within no more than four to four and a half years. Diploma programs, community colleges, and BSN programs must develop articulation agreements that support early completion of a baccalaureate degree program in ways that are feasible, fair, and affordable for all nursing students.

Making the BSN a uniform requirement, however, is not a complete answer to improved patient care. To meet current and near-future practice demands, all nursing programs must upgrade their teaching of nursing science and knowledge; the baccalaureate degree should be but one point on a continuum of degrees and formal learning experiences that include school-to-work transition internships, such as a one-year clinical internship on completion of the first degree, and continuous, career-long learning that includes graduate education for the complex practice of nursing.

We note the promising example of the Oregon Consortium for Nursing Education, an articulated program to allow students to move seamlessly from the community college into a baccalaureate completion program—and beyond. In this new program, students may start their nursing education by earning an associate degree, then directly continue their education to earn a baccalaureate and later a master's degree. In developing the program, the members of the consortium—private and public schools of nursing that grant associate, baccalaureate, and master's degrees—began by considering the nurses Oregonians of the future will need; their design of an articulated system of preparation followed. Moreover, the members of the consortium agreed on the need for new pedagogies and introduced them through comprehensive faculty development and support. The success of the program in forging new ways of preparing nurses highlights the strong value of cooperation for the good of society that we found to be held in high esteem by nursing educators in programs all over the country, a value that could stand nursing education in good stead at this time of crisis.

Licensure

Just as the current system of pathways to nursing practice creates disincentives for entering practice with the BSN, the current standard for licensure is not an incentive for students to seek the BSN. There are no meaningful differences among the NCLEX-RN pass rates of students from the various pathways, even though the large number of test takers can create statistically significant differences. The NCLEX-RN exam uses a mastery scoring system, so test takers need complete only a sufficient number of answers to reach a minimally acceptable pass level. With this type of scoring, absolute numerical differences in total scores are not generated. In most states, students must answer at least 80 percent of the questions correctly. Some states have pegged an acceptable pass at 78 percent.

Finally, it is puzzling that although the national examination for licensure includes many multiple-choice questions on practice, nursing students are not asked to show in simulations their ability to use knowledge for the care of patients, engage in clinical reasoning, or demonstrate ethical comportment. Nursing values highly the ability of its members to practice, yet current licensure exams rely only on comprehensive nursing programs where clinical performance is evaluated. Regulatory assurance of readiness to sit for the licensure requires graduation from an accredited school of nursing where a broader range of evaluation over time occurs.

Addressing the Practice-Education Gap

Neither these structural changes nor others, however, will fully address the practice-education gap unless nursing education makes significant shifts in teaching and curricula. In the next two chapters we describe the faculty and student experience in nursing school and suggest where and how nurse education might build on its considerable strengths to deliver instruction more consistent with the complexities of nursing practice.

2

TEACHING AND LEARNING IN CLINICAL SITUATIONS

IN OUR EFFORT to understand how nursing education prepares students to enter the social contract of the profession, we examined the student experience, augmenting classroom observation and interviews of educators and students with a review of the literature and a national survey of members of the National Student Nurses' Association (NSNA). Of the 32,000 members who had e-mail addresses at the time of the survey, 1,648 responded (a 6 percent response rate). To see the survey instrument, go to www.carnegiefoundation.org/nursing-education/surveys. What emerged, along with particular findings about the student experience, was a view of the points at which the practice-education gap develops. We begin this chapter by looking at teaching and learning in clinical situations. In Chapter Three we examine them inside the classroom and skills labs.

High-Stakes Learning

As soon as students formally enter a nursing program, whether directly as part of community college or a diploma program, or after two years of general education in a baccalaureate program, they begin working with patients, even if it is a mannequin or a fellow student in a simulation lab. They soon enter clinical settings to learn through experience with actual patients in a variety of settings that, over time, range from community sites and patient homes to intensive care. This is what we call experiential learning, or learning from the experience of caring for patients. Students learn from the particular situations of specific patients, which is a hallmark of nursing education and what we refer to as situated learning. Both experiential learning and situated learning are central to nursing education. The student's lay visions of nursing before entering nursing school are often far off the mark, and many students reported being stunned at the high-precision skills and knowledge nurses routinely draw on.

Although the possibility of making a mistake that could lead to the death or injury of a patient is very real and always present, patient safety is enhanced with realistic clinical simulations. Still, high-stakes learning is a necessity; only experiential learning can yield the complex, open-ended, skilled knowledge required for learning to recognize the nature of the particular resources and constraints in equally open-ended and underdetermined clinical situations. Both students and faculty are acutely aware of the dangers of putting learners in the high-risk environment of an acute care hospital. As one student put it: "It is frustrating and scary to function in the clinical setting as an inexperienced student. I often worry that I'll miss something important in a client's condition." Another student captured both the excitement and the weight of responsibility that many other students expressed: "I have had the honor of being present with and learning from clients in intimate, vulnerable, scary situations. I get to regularly advocate for the underserved, especially in the hospital setting. I have access to environments I would have otherwise never been exposed to, and I have learned and grown and broadened my world perspective. I better understand how our system works, and hope someday this knowledge will help me make changes in our system."

Understandably, nursing students fear making a mistake. In interviews and survey responses alike, the student nurses told stories of making mistakes, of reporting their errors, and their terror at the possibility of making a more dangerous error (Rodriguez, 2007). They recognize the level of responsibility of nursing practice, that a nurse's actions could seriously harm the patient or even cause death. The high-stakes experience of the clinical setting makes nursing students aware of the need to actively think about and use their knowledge in the particular situation. If evidence or feedback from a situation does not mesh with their understanding of the situation or interpretation of the information, the student must consider new interpretations, and the clinical teacher uses questions to guide students to search for new interpretations and information.

Learning in Context

Students start their clinical learning in patient care situations that are relatively stable; they are coached and guided as they transfer skills they learned on a mannequin in a skills lab to actual patients, who may be calm or highly anxious, thin or obese, mobile or immobile. As they progress through the program, they are placed in less predictable situations, where the instructors and staff nurses allow them more responsibility and independence in performing tasks, using subtle bedside coaching or more overt coaching outside the patient's room.

A central goal of nursing education is for the learner to develop an attuned, response-based practice and capacity to quickly recognize the nature of whole situations in terms of most pressing and least pressing concerns. As Dewey (1925/1987) suggests, experiential learning does not happen in just any condition, with just any person or on every occasion. Participation in experiential learning requires openness and readiness to improve practice over time, along with clinical reasoning (Dunne, 1993). Experiential learning depends on an environment where feedback on performance is rich and the opportunities for articulating and reflecting on the experiences are deliberately planned.

We found that clinical educators actively give feedback and make full use of the learning opportunities of the clinical situation. Typically, the clinical instructor will prepare the students, as a group, for what they will see and do the next day. During the situation, they coach the students through procedures and use the situation to deepen learning. After the experience, the students and instructor meet in postclinical conference, where the teacher prompts the students to reflect on their experience. Moreover, in the group sessions, students pool their learning, openly sharing their questions and experiences so that their classmates may benefit.

Planning and Feedback

On the night before each clinical assignment, students are expected to do extensive homework related to their assigned patients, to prepare themselves for what they will see and do in the clinical setting the next day. If a student's patient is discharged suddenly or some other change occurs, many clinical instructors will contact their students to give them a new assignment. In preparing for clinical, students review their patient's charts, medications, diagnoses, and complications, and they develop patient care plans for the next day. On the day of care, the students evaluate the plan in the course of care and report any changes or improvements to the plan.

Clinical instructors and students check in with each other throughout the day, the educators making sure that the students are safe and effective as they enter new areas of nursing care. Although we found that nursing students are sometimes placed in the position of observing staff nurses do a procedure, if the clinical instructor is not available the teachers usually coach the student through novel procedures, both outside and inside the patient's room as needed, to ensure accuracy and patient safety. It is worth noting that in contrast, the first- or second-year medical student often shadows the resident or the attending physician, trying to learn through observation and questions about the medical decisions being made with the patients and families.

The nurse educator reassures nursing students that they can go over the procedure before beginning. As one clinical educator noted:

> That's just been a requirement: any new basic procedure, we are with them.... And so they have the opportunity to ask questions, tell us what they're going to do before they go in and do it. At the bedside, I always tell them nursing is part acting, so you always have to act as if you really know what you're doing at the bedside, and if you have any question in the immediate procedure (especially in our group they may freeze, they may have this brain freeze) ... don't hesitate, just ask if we could step out for a moment, outside the room, before you do anything.

The ambiguities of clinical situations are such that practitioners must be organized in their thinking, be able to use their knowledge, and judge when exceptions must be made and when deviations from expectations or the usual are occurring. Clinical instructors model such complex responses for their students. The patient's situation can change rapidly, and invariably the student confronts clinical situations for which she or he is not prepared. The teacher must be open to the possibilities for teaching in each particular clinical situation, as unpredictable and varied as it might be; the teacher looks for the teachable moments, points out what is salient and what needs immediate attention, and helps students integrate and use their knowledge. However, clinical teachers must put patient safety first, at all times. The teacher thus needs to know when to guide the student through questioning and coaching and when to pull the student back and have him observe or assist another nurse, using what Lave and Wenger (1991) call "legitimate peripheral participation," a way to teach students about high-risk situations before they are ready to actually perform in them.

Supporting Learning Through Questions

Many clinical educators engage in on-the-spot assessment of students' understanding and knowledge in the clinical setting, asking students to answer a series of questions that are often posed in rapid succession. As one student explained, "They draw out of you what you know: 'A prudent nurse would, dot, dot, dot, fill in the blank. This medication is for? And why are you giving it? And in the medication scheme of things, what is the most important? They're having dialysis in an hour.' [If I say,] 'My patient is having dialysis,' [the teacher asks] '*What if* they also had heart failure?' The faculty person still wants you to answer the 'what if' question. . . . I have a profound appreciation for these questioning sessions and finding out what I don't know."

Clinical educators typically use what-if questions to help students extend their thinking about a clinical situation, about the ramifications of potential changes and differences in their patients. One educator explained, "I think we all use a lot of 'what if' questions: 'What if this happens, what if that happens, what if the client did that?'" For example, one teacher described a role-playing activity: "And we all get to be different people. . . . I got to be a sixty-five-year-old male last week and I was also a fourteen-year-old female. And then the group member behaves like the fourteen-year-old female or the sixty-five-year-old male and asks us questions." Another teacher talked about "the what-if game" that she uses in both classroom and clinical:

> I like to throw out a lot of questions like this: "What do you think if, what would be different if . . . ?" So the student will tell me a little bit about the patient and I'll say, "What if the patient were fifty, what if the patient had hypertension, what if the patient told you that right this minute she had chest pain? What would you do?" So that's the what-if game . . . . In clinical they love it, they actually love it. "Ask me another question": I've actually had my students say that to me. "Oh, don't go, ask me another question."

Asking students to think about what would happen to their patients if something in their situation was different encourages the student to think about similar patients in varying circumstances, or similar circumstances with different patients. Faculty draw on other questioning strategies, as this student explained:

> I had a patient who had a Whipple surgical procedure. I had just received the patient from surgery and I'd done some pre-clinical work on it and my clinical instructor said, "Well, what are your top three nursing diagnoses for this patient?" That put me right on the spot. Right when I first picked up the patient and just did an initial assessment and had to go over his first . . . I had maybe fifteen minutes and two-thirds of his medications had to be given at nine o'clock. But rather than being in gear for the meds, I had to be in gear for, "OK, what's the bigger picture, why he's being given these meds, what are

we trying to do in these first hours post-operatively?" Your head is so
filled up with things you've got to do, you don't necessarily take the
overall and bigger picture in a clinical setting and [the] clinical instructor is hitting you right away with, "OK, what is it we're trying to do
here?" That kind of questioning is really important.

Another student commented, "I find it very useful that [my clinical
instructor] comes to the floor and asks those questions. I find that it
engages me in a way that I'm going to think about." As another student
explained, "And it's not that they're doing it because they don't trust us,
you know; it's not like they're peering over our shoulders. . . . You know,
maybe the first couple of weeks we were there, they wanted to make sure
but now, they do trust us, but they also are very conscientious to check to
make sure that we're doing it right. Or before we do a procedure, they'll
ask us, "What are you going to do? When you go in there what are you
going to do? Walk me through it step by step."

As students progress through the program, the clinical teacher helps the
student examine the patient's context to help her see the whole situation,
asking such questions such as, "What does this patient need most? Fear
most?" and "What are the patient's most significant concerns in terms
of their family and everyday life?" Clinical teachers will ask advanced
students to compare new clinical situations with prior ones, or imagine a
different patient.

Developing Clinical Reasoning and Judgment

Clinical reasoning is the ability to reason about a clinical situation as
it unfolds, as well as about patient and family concerns and context.
It always calls for understanding the temporal nature of a case. Good
nursing judgments can also never ignore the concerns and "lifeworld" of
the injured or ill patient.

We observed that many clinical educators use pedagogies of contextualization, whereby they usher student nurses into a practice in which
the nurse is always present for the unique patient in the situation as it
unfolds while also remaining aware of what has gone before. *Contextualization* means taking into account the response of the particular patient
in the situation, including the patient's history, interrelationships between
physiological systems, social interactions with others, and responses to
the particular environment. Nurses confront multiple levels of context,
from physiology to the family and social world of the patient.

Students come into the clinical setting with assessment skills they have tried to learn in a skills lab. Clinical educators often try to help the students translate these skills from the static lab environment to the dynamic patient care environment by pointing out relevant information and guiding the student to pay attention in order to contextualize their assessment of the patient as they care for them. Some clinical educators weave context into teaching procedures, which may be as simple as giving an injection to a patient:

> You teach them to perform a new skill in a nurturing environment, so that no question is stupid; and then to move them from the point of taking the cap off the needle without contaminating it, to being able to identify an injection site, using anatomical landmarks; deliver medication; get that needle back out and dispose of it without sticking yourself. Then the student is guided to look at the response of the patient. So that whole thing of being able to help students to think about not only "Do I need to assess the patient and see why they need a pain med?" [but also] "I have to get the correct pain med and do the six rights of pain medication administration. Then I go and deliver it and then I have to make sure that I follow up and see if it was effective." And it has to be in the context of the patient. It cannot be in the context of a task alone.

This teacher articulates how good nursing practice always connects skillful performance of a task with the skill of attunement to the patient's experience and concern. Pedagogies of contextualization include teaching students to avoid overgeneralization from a situation or stereotyping of patients. Instead, they include situated teaching and coaching to help students take into account the patient's unique history in evaluating signs and symptoms:

> We were caring for a diabetic patient who had a low blood sugar that morning and they had done interventions to bring the blood sugar back up. The student got there two hours later. She came to me and said, "He doesn't look right, he's kind of pale." And I said, "Is he sweating?" She said, "Yes," so I said, "Well, what do you think is going on here? What do you think we ought to do?" We talked through it. If he had low blood sugar two hours ago, and they didn't recheck it, then maybe it's still low. And if he's pale and he's sweaty, then that means more than likely it is low. And it was low, 47 [normal fasting is 70-99]. So then we had to do some interventions. The thing is that the primary nurse had been in there and didn't catch it. So it was a learning experience not only for the student but for the staff nurse, who was a fairly new nurse.

Pedagogies of Contextualization

Students must learn to put their patients' experience into context, including the cultural background, the patient's environment, illness experience, and relationships with the patient and the family. For example, a clinical educator explained how she uses patient assessment to throw light on the situation a patient is in: "In my view, it's being aware of the surroundings of a patient, of their behaviors. To me assessment is not necessarily just physical assessment, which we also do. You know, listen[ing] to [their] heart and lungs and doing all of those, but you also assess the client's interactions. In obstetrics, I assess interactions with their infant, interactions between them and their spouse. I think assessment requires an awareness of the whole surrounding that the client's in."

Nurses expect to coach patients and family members on coping and managing their illness or injury. Nurses are taught to consider the patient's physical environment, the nature of their social and care support, and how patients view their health and illness. Patients recover, but their recovery is not limited to the physiological system. Effective and useful nursing assessment must consider a broader view than a review of physiology. The best nurse's assessment is contextualized, as this faculty member noted:

> I teach a lot of the "Specific Course" lab and it's a good opportunity to start teaching them about assessing the patient's environment. For instance, when we're going to a community clinic and someone's coming in the door and I tell them, "Watch that person come toward you and you can gather a tremendous amount of information without even asking; just by watching how they walk, how they carry themselves, those kinds of things. So you get into the habit of looking at your people and touching them as well. The warmth of the skin can tell you a lot. Plus it's comforting to most people to have a touch." So, we start there.

Nurses must quickly learn that knowing *what* and *how* is not enough; they must also know *when*. We found that clinical educators coach students to develop clinical judgment by having them focus on setting priorities. In fast-paced complex clinical environments, nurses and physicians must know which things it is more important to do first. Priority setting has to be plastic, stretching and bending to fit rapidly changing situations. With expertise, nurses learn to respond fluidly to each situation's demands (Benner, 2000; Benner et al., 2009). This fluidity is possible through the experience of reading situations and responding to changes. We found that the clinical learning experience helps students develop these core skills that contribute to a sense of salience in order to grasp what is most important for a particular patient.

Setting Priorities

For the novice, the beginning nursing student, the obstacle to setting priorities is that all tasks, requests, and concerns seem to be of equal weight; they must all be done (Benner, 2005; Benner et al., 2009). At first, figuring out which tasks are more urgent requires deliberate thought because the student has not yet learned to see the big picture or gained a tacit sense of salience that makes some things stand out as more or less important. A faculty member described teaching students trying to gain this sense of salience:

> It seems like when they first come to you they are so task-oriented, so focused on, "I've got to give my meds at 10:00 A.M.," without the picture that Mr. Smith is having chest pain down the hall, so those 10:00 A.M. meds are not as important right now. Once they get to that senior level and they're working with a preceptor, then it's more about the big picture: "How am I going to manage all four of these patients and all four of their needs right now?" I try to teach them time management and how they're going to handle all these things happening at one time in their senior clinical assignments. And it goes back to autonomy, because they have to have the confidence to make those decisions: "OK, do I go help Ms. So-and-so get on the bedpan, or do I need to go see about the chest pain?" And to me that's so simple, but they'll spend a lot of time figuring out what to do first ... and it's so interesting to watch them in the beginning. I used to say, "She's circling, she's circling."

A student describes gaining a sense of salience and setting priorities: "Prioritizing is something that we learned right away, and I mean day one. They say, 'You want to make sure you prioritize which things you want to do first, second, third.' We talk about that through every course, and through every disease process. What symptoms pop up first and how to deal with them right away ... if you are doing your assessment, you have to know what's important. If you run across a problem—for example, they have a few crackles in their lungs, but they have a really irregular heart rhythm—which is more important?" Another student describes how her clinical teachers help her learn. "And our instructors, I think are really good in the clinical setting ... if we're on medical-surgical floor, they're really good at, 'OK, this is what your problem is: What are you going to do first? What should we get done first? Which one takes importance and then where do you go from there?'"

We found that in clinical settings, students develop clinical judgment through coaching about priorities. Through this coaching, students learn that most patient care goals are important, but not equally urgent. The challenge is greater for the beginning student when she still experiences competing tasks as having a similar level of urgency. Planning and priority setting offer faculty a context for helping students develop their clinical judgment in specific situations, as this faculty member noted:

> You start by being right there with the student as they're looking over the chart, as they're looking over the patient's history, as they're looking over their meds, as they're planning for their day. I talk to them about what's a priority, ask them, "What do you need to do first?" For example, if the person had just had surgery the day before and needs to be up and walking. [I say,] "What are you going to do before you get them up to walk? Do they need some pain medications?" . . . [T]he first time you do some of these things it's more modeling for the students, and you need to be there with them to kind of guide them and say, "Well, maybe instead of doing this activity first, it would be better to back up and do this first. I mean you don't want to get him up to walk right after he's just had something for pain. You need to let that work for a little while and then get him up." So then I ask, "How long does it take for the medication you just gave to act? When is it at its height of effectiveness for that patient?" and then work from there. And as they progress through the clinical rotations, then you can see growth and see how the modeling has helped them look beyond just what they are doing right at that very moment.

Setting priorities—or "prioritizing," as nurse educators call it—focuses on ordering one's interventions and nursing care by first assessing and discerning the nature of the situation. However, because priorities constantly shift, clinical educators teach with an eye to change, and the changing relevance of the patient care goals as the patient's clinical and psychosocial issues change. With repeated experiences of setting priorities, students develop a sense of salience. Urgent issues that are obvious become part of the student's sense of salience, allowing him to notice what must be addressed immediately without necessarily "setting priorities." In the beginning, the student must pay attention and deliberately set priorities, with experience developing a sense of salience and along with it allowing the student to *notice* urgent issues in a clinical situation. This allows the practitioner to learn more nuanced appraisals of new situations, focusing on what is puzzling or unusual.

Priorities, once set, are typically not viewed as stable, as this faculty member illustrates:

> Lately we've started our morning with a conference and each student has been asked to identify what they think their priority of care is going to be for that day based on what they've done as far as their preparation and looking up everything about that client. And then we come to [postclinical] conference and we say, "This was your priority. Did it turn out that way?" And we spend part of the time talking about what changed about the client. And we have one student whose client the day before was extremely upset. They had done a biopsy and found widespread prostate cancer. And come the next day, they had done further testing and found that it wasn't so widespread. So the client was overjoyed and the student was pleased to change her care plan that had initially intended to allow the patient to talk about his terminal illness, or express anticipatory grieving. And so we talked about how you need to be aware of changes and be able to change gears rather quickly.

The clinical educator stresses the importance of both developing a plan as part of preclinical preparation and also being flexible and open to change. It underlines the need for students to be flexible in the face of nursing practice, where nurses must set priorities in order to act in an environment of multiple patient assignments and multiple demands on their time and attention. Priority setting has to be fluid and efficient because the clinical environment and patients' conditions change rapidly.

A teacher described how her program structures clinical assignments by assigning two patients instead of one, using the increased demands as a way to help the student learn how make decisions about what must be done first:

> I sort of force them into decision making when I assign them two patients and they have to decide what needs to get done. But they have to actually plan what they intend to do, and then, we all know, sometimes these plans change, and what they thought they were going to do at 7:30 changes dramatically and they have to be flexible enough and adaptable enough to think on their feet, pull in all the knowledge base and experiential base they have at that point and adjust the plan and then evaluate what they've done and see how well that plan is working and, if not, they have to move on to another plan.

A Missed Opportunity

As effective as the coaching on priorities might be, however, overall we found little formal instruction on *how* to set priorities. Few rules or other abstract guidelines were offered. The bulk of the teaching and learning about selecting the most important priorities occurred in specific clinical settings and referred to particular patients. Flexibility and adaptability were emphasized to help students change their priorities as the patient's concerns and needs changed.

We further found that students struggle to develop a sense of salience. As one faculty member put it:

> In this particular class, they tend to struggle most in terms of being prepared for clinical and walking through, "These are my patient's problems." I think it's just due to lack of experience and the complexity of the patients that they have to care for, which we have no control over, because the patients are so sick. "OK, now I want you to identify your patient's top three priorities." I don't think students in the beginning have a good concept of what prioritizing problems really is like. You know, what it really entails. They have a lot of difficulty with that.

Priority setting is an important educational goal, and we question whether the process of setting priorities for a menu of interventions for particular patients is addressed sufficiently, even in clinical settings. The situated questioning and coaching in the clinical setting is useful and highly valued by students and educators alike, but its focus is often abstract: "What assessments and interventions in general are used for patients of this general type?" A number of educators mentioned that, if no major inconvenience or harm might be caused to either learner or patient, they intentionally let a student proceed with a plan of care that may not work well. In this way, they help the student learn to read the situation and evaluate the impact of their planning and interventions. This seems a roundabout way of teaching, and it precludes opportunities for the student to work through more complex, high-risk situations. We also noted that setting priorities is not addressed in the classroom, where educators *could* focus on the more general problem of how to set priorities in the context of teaching about a disease process or clinical condition, and coach students on priority setting through presentation of clinical vignettes. Doing so would contribute to developing students' sense of salience. More focus on *identifying* relevant concerns in the classroom would strengthen the students' intellectual skill of setting priorities in the clinical setting. Indeed, we found missing in most classroom teaching an explicit focus on patient care assessments, evaluating treatment goals in relation to the patient's condition and concerns, and identifying the interventions and setting priorities for the most urgent needs.

What might be more effective is to give students the opportunity and time in the classroom to rehearse priority setting for specific patients. Here students can safely make mistakes and work through the process of arriving at the most important actions to take with particular patients. As an example, we point to the classroom strategy described in Part Three, where the classroom teacher effectively uses questions about patient assessment and identification of patient care interventions in the course of an unfolding case about a specific patient.

Developing a Rationale

Although nursing students receive little formal instruction on setting priorities, they are explicitly expected to develop rationales as they set priorities for any patient care intervention, thus linking prioritizing with having a rationale for the chosen actions and their order. This requirement for students to draw on nursing knowledge to justify their actions is pervasive in nursing education. Increasingly, in acute care settings, therapies and medications are titrated or adjusted according to the patient's physiological responses; this requires the nurse's ongoing attention and reaction to patients' physiological responses. Students were clear that they had to have a rationale for what they were doing, and that they were expected to actively solve problems amid changing clinical situations. They explained how clinical educators model this:

STUDENT 1: And then if we do something that's not what they would do, they'd explain what they would do first and give us a rationale of why they would do that first besides something else.

STUDENT 2: Rationale is a big part of that.

STUDENT 1: And I think our instructors are really good about always telling us why. It's not "This is this way because I said it's this way."

STUDENT 3: They always give us a good reason on why they do the things that they do.

Some students noted that at first it seemed strange that their instructors always asked why and wanted a clearly thought out rationale, but supplying a rationale has become "just automatic." Teaching students to be able to defend their actions with a verbal explanation is in part born of the hierarchical arrangement in medical care; nurses have little authority but a great deal of responsibility and must justify their actions to patients and families, physicians, other nurses, and administrators. Although the focus on rationale may reflect nurses' lower status, being able to state one's rationale is a good way to check for faulty assumptions, or a mistaken grasp of the nature of the clinical situation. Being clear in one's thinking about rationale before acting contributes to increasing safety in the high-stakes environment of acute care. For example, safety engineers recommend verbalizing one's assumptions and rationale while acting in rapidly changing dangerous situations, such as fighting a wildfire, in order to detect faulty thinking and inappropriate actions (Weick & Sutcliffe, 2001). The clinical educators' insistence on requiring students to verbalize the rationale for their actions is an important step in internalizing this kind of thinking for practice.

Learning How to Act in the Situation

Nursing education stands out from other professions in its emphasis in clinical practice on knowing what, how, and when. Nurse educators emphasize how important it is for students to understand the rationale for their actions, and the next level of expertise: knowing how to take all the steps necessary for action. To take action in a given patient care situation, the nurse must have a fluent grasp of the relevant medical information and be able to translate it into practical knowledge.

For example, one teacher told us about coaching a student who was taking care of a patient receiving morphine. When the teacher asked the student, "If the patient were given too much morphine, what signs and symptoms should you be aware of?" the student answered correctly (decreased responsiveness and lower respiration), adding that the patient would need Narcan, a drug to reverse the effects of the morphine. The teacher, however, was not finished; she asked the student where the Narcan was kept. The student answered correctly that it was in a locked cabinet, and the teacher waited, finally asking the student where to find the key. In this example, the teacher's questions guided the student to think about a whole host of concerns if the patient experienced an overdose: to note and interpret the changes in the patient's breathing, color, and overall appearance; to decide on the appropriate drug and action to reverse the effects of the morphine; and then to be able to carry out that action—in this case quickly, if need be.

Clinical Reasoning-in-Transition

Clinical situations are open-ended. In a given situation many trajectories or trends are possible, making clinical situations underdetermined. Unlike classroom descriptions of disease in which diagnostic criteria and associated laboratory values are clear and objectively defined, human beings present with several diseases at once in ways that defy the objective and rational deductive thought processes too often modeled and valued in the classroom. Thus, caring for individual patients requires that the nurse use a form of practical reasoning that we have come to describe as *clinical reasoning-in-transition* (Benner, Hooper-Kyriakidis, & Stannard, 1999). This form of reasoning keeps track of the particular patient, how the illness or illnesses are unfolding, and the meaning of the patient's responses. It requires keeping track of a narrative of what has been tried and what has or has not worked with the patient. Clinical reasoning-in-transition requires from the clinician a thoughtful stance of attentiveness, respect, curiosity, inquiry, and willingness to be "pulled up short" in her thinking, all framed by the clinician's concern for the good of the patient (Gadamer, 1975; Kerdeman, 2004). Kerdeman (2004) points out that the prevailing view of "reflective learning" assumes that self-questioning and challenging one's assumptions and prejudgments are activities that students can and should be taught to do purposively. However, Kerdeman argues, sometimes our understanding is thrown into question without our deliberate attention: "This particular experience of negation is what Gadamer means by being pulled up short. When we are pulled up short, events we neither want nor foresee and to which we may believe we are immune, interrupt our lives and challenge our self-understanding in ways that are painful but transforming" (2004, p. 145). In situations of care where clinicians are brought up short, the clinical situation prevails over the clinician, "comes and finds us out" (p. 151), and interrupts a clinician's taken-for-granted understandings and assumptions. However, the experience of being brought up short has another requirement. We can be transformed by these experiences only when we allow ourselves to notice and acknowledge the misunderstandings that we might prefer to ignore.

By encouraging students to allow themselves to be brought up short, teachers help students form a moral disposition that will foster a self-improving practice. Sometimes students have difficulty staying open in their reasoning about a patient's situation. They may get stuck on one particular aspect of the patient's situation. For example, a faculty member reported that a fourteen-year-old patient was admitted for vomiting and diarrhea. When the nursing assistant tried to get the patient up for a weight check, the patient became dizzy and fell down, hitting her head. The patient was not badly injured, but an incident report had to be filled out. The student nurse became focused on the incident report and who was responsible for the fall. This teacher explains that her goal was to redirect the student's thinking:

> Well, what is the important issue here? Is the important issue to put a finger on whoever is weighing the child and who is responsible for the patient's fall? Or is it to figure out what is going on with this patient? And so I got the student through a series of questions to think about what possibly might be going on with the patient: 'Why might the patient be dizzy? Why might the patient have fallen?' And thinking about dehydration: 'Okay, what else could we assess on this patient?' And to make a long story short, the patient ended up getting some IV boluses and started getting back on track. I was trying to move the student from thinking about just one piece of that event to getting a better understanding of what was going on, and thinking about the focus. But it took quite a few questions.

As the clinical educator redirects the student's thinking to her patient, she helps her student develop a sense of salience about what is most important in this situation, reminding the student that the focus on the patient's well-being must be primary, and not the incident report, or assigning blame in the incident. The teacher coached her student in using reasoning-in-transition by focusing her on context and sequencing her actions. The teacher also gently pushed the student to allow herself to be brought up short, to reconsider her focus on the incident report and laying blame.

Learning to Respond to Changes in the Patient's Condition

Because the patients' condition changes and because it is the nurse who is on the front line, spending the most time with the patient, a crucial part of nursing practice is detecting these changes and adjusting nursing care as well as alerting the physician about patient changes in order to prompt changes in medical treatments. Clinical educators coached students to stay open to the possibility that a situation may call for changes. This kind of coaching helps to instill in students the disposition for being open to being brought up short as exemplified in this exchange:

> I bring the case to the student so that we can work through the questions: So what would you do next? So this patient isn't fitting the profile. We don't want to give students blueprints but have them adjust

their care to go along with the person's current developmental stage, to go along with the cultural concerns of the patient, what they normally eat. So we teach the student to think in a lot of different directions instead of putting things in boxes most of the time ... [We ask], "This is the patient, this happens, what do you do next?" And they *can't* look at their notes and memorize how to answer the question.

Clinical reasoning involves assessing the immediate history in order to account for changes in the patient's current condition, combined with reasoning across real-time transitions as the patient's condition and concerns continue to evolve. Clinical educators put much effort into teaching students the importance of ongoing assessment over time with attention to what is different *now*. By drawing the student's attention to the shortcomings of a plan made the night before, for example, the teacher helps the student learn how to think in a changing situation. Teachers need to achieve an important balance in these coaching situations, as they negotiate the tension between helping students feel they are mastering the practice while at the same time encouraging students to stay open to what is unknown and unforeseen, or to having their assumptions and misunderstandings turned around when needed.

Detective Work

We frequently observed clinical educators using teaching strategies that help students develop reasoning-in-transition skills. For instance, we found that some clinical educators deliberately teach their students to engage in "detective work" by giving them the daily clinical assignment of "sleuthing" for undetected drug incompatibilities, questionable drug dosages, and unnoticed signs and symptoms. For example, one student noted that an unusual dosage of a heart medication was being given to a patient who did not have heart disease. She first asked her teacher about the unusually high dosage. The teacher, in turn, asked the student whether she had asked the patient's staff nurse or the patient about the dosage. The nurse did not know why the patient was receiving the high dosage and assumed it was for heart disease; she had not questioned the order. When the student asked the patient, the student found that the medication was being given for tremors; the patient and the doctor had titrated the dosage for control of the tremors.

Deliberately teaching detective work is similar to teaching "critical reflection" but keeps the student situated and engaged, ferreting out the immediate history and unfolding of events. In that respect, this pedagogical strategy teaches *modus operandi thinking*, a form of clinical or practical reasoning-in-transition that most resembles criminal detective work, trying to figure out the patterns in an open, puzzling situation of crime. In nursing practice, the nurse tries to figure out what the patient's particular ordering and nature of trends of vital signs and signs and symptoms means. As one student told us, her greatest reward in nursing education is "using skills learned in classroom and lab settings; connecting pathophysiology with real patients; putting the puzzle together."

Many nurse educators expect students to figure out the patient's illness and hospitalization trajectory from reading the patient record. However, the record is not as straightforward as it might seem. A student may determine, in preclinical planning, that the patient's trajectory is headed toward point A, but when he encounters the patient the next day, he must think about what has changed since the day before and whether the patient's condition still fits the trajectory for which he had planned. Because it is often the case that the patient's condition does not, discovering this requires the student to reason-in-transition. As one educator describes, sometimes it takes some detective work just to figure out why the patient is still in the hospital:

> The student didn't recognize that seven days was too long for a patient with an appendectomy to be in the hospital and that's experience. "Let's go look at the patient and let's take a little bit better history. Did you hear anything in report?" Of course, there was nothing in report because the report's not as thorough as it should be. So we had to do a little detective work to find out that the patient actually had gangrene in his colon and that's why he was there seven days later.

Central to clinical reasoning-in-transition is the ability to recognize subtle changes in a patient's condition over time. Most hospital therapies and diagnoses require that the nurse evaluate the patient's responses to therapies and tests and, when ordered, make adjustments to the patient's therapies accordingly. For example, nurses evaluate patient responses and titrate vaso-active drugs or analgesia and sedation. As one nurse educator related, she met a student's reluctance to recognize that the patient's condition was deteriorating by introducing detective work:

> [The] patient was supposedly stable [yet] was actually rapidly deteriorating. I saw this but the staff nurse responsible for the patient did not see it. And the student was really wanting to be a *real nurse* and identified with the staff nurse who was saying, "I can tolerate these changes, these things happen, everything is fine." And I kept saying,

"Everything is *not* fine. This patient needs to go to the ICU." And so I had to make that student become engaged with this problem and then I said, "OK, let's think of one test we could do that would really demonstrate to us that this patient is deteriorating rapidly." And so we agreed that it would be the blood gasses. And we had to do this very quickly. And if the patient were fine we would find blood gasses this way, if not we would find it this way. And I knew I was right; I knew that the blood gasses would demonstrate that the patient was not fine. We got an order to have the blood gasses taken and of course, I was right. The patient was in the ICU right away.

One nurse's perception and hunch were verified with lab work—in this case, blood gasses—while another nurse's hunch was disconfirmed. The teacher knew that her hunch would be confirmed by the blood gasses report and in the process the student would learn about the effectiveness of reasoning-in-transition. Holding tightly to a gut feeling without further investigation is unacceptable, but following through the reasoning process by engaging in "if-then" forms of reasoning to confirm or disconfirm the hunch is good practice. Although if-then reasoning generally requires a deep background understanding of the particular clinical situation and relevant science in order to come up with the right questions (this educator knew that the blood glasses would answer the question faster and more definitively than a countless array of other possible diagnostic tests), the teacher took the opportunity to model for the student thinking like a nurse by formulating appropriate questions.

Challenges to Clinical Teaching

The challenges to clinical teaching are many, ranging from supply of placements and preceptors to coordination with classroom learning. Some challenges are simply a matter of being in the health care environment. By the very nature of the practice for which they are teaching, the extent to which nurse educators can design or control the students' experiential learning has limits; among other things, mixed messages abound. Students hear about the importance of considering patients' personal and social lives, their stress, their coping, and their suffering. In their clinical rotations, however, many find these issues unattended to, even unarticulated, in our health care system. For example, students might study the social causes of family violence and the need to address family violence in the emergency room; yet in the actual emergency care setting they often find the focus is primarily on the physical care of the patient and the legal issues of the incident. In formal classroom teaching, attention to relational practices is all but excluded, having been pushed out by a narrow technical focus and a predominant emphasis on classification and cataloguing of medical and nursing knowledge.

On the surveys we conducted in collaboration with AACN and NLN and in faculty interviews, clinical educators report that finding and maintaining good clinical sites is a major challenge. One described her experience as "always a challenge to find instructors and sites ... All the hospitals have different requirements for students and instructors." Some reported that the student-instructor ratio was skewed, which made it difficult to teach well. One noted that the biggest challenge was the clinical group size: "We consistently have groups of eight to ten sophomore or entry-level nursing students. We don't have adequate time to spend with them to ensure they are learning all the concepts. It is too focused on obtaining or performing the skills. Also, there is a safety issue when passing medication with this many students. Nurses on the clinical unit would not be assigned this many patients!"

Another clinical instructor sketched the difficulties she had with "correlating what the students are learning in class and trying to present similar situations or experiences in clinical to supplement their learning and make it more meaningful. Very time-intensive on my part, but I feel that it is what I should be doing to help students learn."

Some among those who teach in both settings remarked that their schools do not acknowledge the amount of work demanded of nursing educators. Faculty interviews and surveys contained many comments similar to this educator's observation:

> The teaching and clinical workloads are extremely heavy. Nursing courses, especially clinical courses, differ from most other courses taught at our university. It is difficult for us to communicate with administrators how the clinical aspect of nursing is different from other courses. At our university, load credit is calculated based on in-class course and lab courses. The ratio used for lab courses is the same ratio used for our clinical courses. A general lab class on campus is very different from taking students into the hospital to provide care. Using this formula results in very heavy course loads for our nursing faculty. Additionally the ratio of having ten students per one teacher is too high, even for experienced teachers in student-friendly agencies. Our state board of nursing and many of our agencies know the ten-to-one ratio is too high but no one has been willing to take the bold step of changing the ratio to seven-to-one or maximum eight-to-one.

I encourage our state boards of nursing and nursing accrediting bodies
to reexamine their position on this important nursing issue.

This nurse educator points out that effectively teaching and supervising
ten students in a clinical setting is nearly impossible, and often hazardous.
However, other educators who have no clinical teaching assignment may
find it difficult to imagine the intensity of clinical teaching, and therefore
school policy may not give adequate teaching credit for clinical teaching. We suggest that, in programs where this is the case, academic deans
shadow nurse educators during their clinical teaching in order to understand the full extent of their work. This is an important point; faculty
work overload is a crucial problem in recruitment and retention of nurse
faculty.

The students also described challenges to learning in the clinical setting.
One student explained the experience of moving from one clinical site to
another: "We are constantly being rotated through different units. As soon
as we have been on the unit long enough to get the hang of things, we
rotate to a new unit or hospital. Each hospital uses different equipment
and a different charting system. Also, preceptors can greatly differ in how
they do things. So if you do something the way a previous preceptor
teaches you, the next preceptor may say that it is wrong."

In the survey and interviews, students also reported feeling "blind-
sided" because they could not predict how they would be received by
staff nurses. When the students arrive on site, especially if they are beginning a new clinical rotation, they often have little information about the
nurses with whom they will work side by side. Students were uneasy about
what to expect from clinical instructors. One commented, "Depending
on which clinical instructor you get, you may use no classroom content in
the clinical placement or you may constantly use classroom content in the
clinical site. It all depends on the luck of the draw and which clinical
instructor you get. There is no streamlined system where all of the
clinical instructors do the same thing."

We found that the teaching and coaching by school-based clinical educators was generally more effective and integrative than that by staff
nurses assigned to teach students. Partnering staff nurse teachers often
receive no guidance or have no learning opportunities in teaching, much
less in achieving the objectives of the particular course. Yet staff nurses
are essential to the clinical education of student nurses. Student accounts
of their experiences with nurses at clinical sites varied widely. Some students found nurses they wanted to emulate. As one put it, "The nurse
I was assigned to was a wonderful role model. I know what to shoot

for." Another student appreciated "getting to work with some wonderful nurses in the hospital who take the time and have the patience to do one-on-one teaching ... and under their guidance, feeling like I have something worthwhile to offer the patients." Another described excellent clinical instruction as "having a great nurse that will teach you so much while you are in your clinical rotation. One that is willing to let you do everything while she watches so that you get the experience."

However, many students reported that they had difficulties working side by side with staff nurses. One noted, "The most difficult thing for me is to gain good knowledge and practice at the hospital setting when some of the nurses who precept me do not want to help me. It is discouraging to see that nurses sometimes see me just as an extra pair of hands rather than as a student who still needs help and has questions." Another student remarked, "At times we are treated as an inconvenience to them. In my opinion, becoming a nurse means that you must sometimes assume the role of a teacher. Many of the nurses out in the work force lack the drive it takes to mentor and teach aspiring nurses. This includes some of the charge nurses I have come in contact with, who act like they do not have the time to 'deal' with a student."

Still other students expressed dismay at attitudes of staff nurses toward student nurses. One student called it "horizontal violence," saying, "Nurses love to eat their young! If the staff nurses could realize we are there to learn, it would help. Nasty comments help no one. It's difficult to learn while walking on eggshells." Another student related, "Sometimes the nurses are rude to us nursing students, and this is very discouraging. During this last summer, I had one preceptor who was very rude to me during the entire shift, and she even yelled at me at one point. Needless to say, this made me not want to work at that particular hospital anymore, and I switched hospitals." Summarizing what she learned, another student observed, "With the nurses who are not so kind, or even quite hateful to students, it shows me how not to be." When most students enter a clinical setting, it is often unfamiliar territory to them as a place to learn. They may meet nurses who accept them whole-heartedly and see them as future colleagues or others who express outright hostility. In the next chapter we discuss teaching and learning in a setting far more familiar to all students: the classroom.

3

TEACHING AND LEARNING IN THE CLASSROOM AND SKILLS LAB

NURSING EDUCATION is sharply divided by location. Students and faculty alike discussed learning and teaching in clinical and classroom settings, including skills laboratories, as though they were entirely different from each other. For example, many students referred to what they learned in the classroom as "theory" that they then "applied" in clinical settings, implying that the nursing knowledge taught in classrooms is important but somehow different from the nursing knowledge students learn in clinical settings. It also suggests separation of learning and experiences, with theory being delivered in lectures and applied knowledge being gained through clinical situations. This terminology reflects a significant problem in nursing education, one we address throughout this book: the expectation that clinical and classroom teaching and learning will be separate and a narrow rational-technical approach is sufficient for using knowledge in practice. By "a narrow rational-technical approach" here we mean the assumption that a student in a clinical situation can learn formal criteria or decision rules for complex clinical situations with no adjustment for the variations in the situation. For example, even for advanced clinical life support (ACLS) rules, which are generally correct, a patient's reaction to particular drugs, or particular cardiac pathophysiology or hemodynamic condition, may call for alterations in the ACLS. If the patient's history is especially well known to the clinicians, there are usually exceptions or changes made.

One student explained that because of the division of learning into clinical and classroom settings, it is "difficult to get the full picture and understand the pathophysiology behind the disease processes. And without the background knowledge, I wouldn't understand why I performed a task or how to explain the situation to a patient." Although clinical and classroom learning does of course occur in differing settings, often taught by different teachers, students were expected to somehow integrate the parts into a whole.

As revealed in both student interviews and comments on the survey, students are distressed at the quality of teaching and learning in classrooms and skill labs and the lack of patient care simulations. A student who responded to the Carnegie-NSNA survey said that one of the biggest challenges in nursing education she faced was "being lectured on caring and building trust by instructors who don't practice what they preach ... learning from instructors who may be great nurses, but haven't received training in teaching and communicating effectively as lecturers."

Many students reported similar experiences with lecturers and lectures, and their responses consistently revealed uneasiness with how faculty lectured and the amount of information in their lectures, as well as the heavy reliance on such presentation tools as Microsoft PowerPoint. One talked about realizing how disengaged she was: "It's really easy to sit there and agree with everything that [teachers are] saying and then an hour later if you try and recall it, you're kind of hazy on what it was because you just don't retain it when you just sit there and you watch these slides go by. And it got to the point where some of us stopped printing the slides and we'd just sit there and try to take notes. And we were learning better, but the problem was, they were going too fast." Another student remarked, "there have to be other ways to get the information needed to be a nurse without being overloaded and relying on just memorization to pass a class. Remembering this information is important, memorization does help to a certain extent, but it doesn't mean a student really understands the entire concept." Indeed, a 2003 Institute of Medicine report warns of the many problems that arise when educators expect their students to rely too much on memory (Greiner & Knebel, 2003). Student nurses see problems with teaching and learning in terms of compromising or jeopardizing their ability to administer safe and effective patient care. They pointed out, in site visits and in the Carnegie-NSNA surveys, that they need more connections between what is taught in the classroom and their clinical experiences.

Teaching and Learning—Removed from Practice

As observers, we too were distressed at the approach to teaching in the nursing classroom. Experiential learning is one of the strengths of nursing education; we found a sharp contrast between the classroom situation, where it was for the most part absent, and clinical situations, where it is common. Teachers in classrooms often rely heavily on automated presentation software and use pedagogical strategies that are significantly less effective than teachers generally use in clinical settings and skills labs, where knowledge acquisition and use are more integrated. Although we note and applaud the exceptions to this finding, classroom teachers who make an effort to integrate the classroom and clinical experiences, and the even fewer who make the classroom a setting for rich, experiential learning, the research team was struck by the variability and even poor quality of teaching in classrooms and skill and simulation laboratories. This situation has grave implications for the extent to which students will develop skills of clinical inquiry and the ability to use knowledge in specific clinical situations.

In addition to classroom teaching, nurse educators also rely on skills laboratories, where they can demonstrate nursing practice outside the clinical setting. Skills laboratories are an intermediate zone between the classroom, where students learn nursing knowledge, and the clinical setting, where students learn to use that knowledge when caring for patients. In the skills lab, students can practice with equipment and technology or undertake simulation exercises that attempt to mimic practice and integrate knowledge acquisition and knowledge use.

In ticking off a list of things that overwhelm her and her colleagues, one educator summed up comments we heard: "The difficulty in recruiting more instructors, the very long hours, the very short pay, the change in textbooks, the need to continually improve and update our own knowledge of nursing while staying current with technology and improving teaching techniques, continual work toward maintaining accreditation, preparation for coursework each semester, and clinical prep and evaluation, the unrest in nursing, and the feeling that I am 'throwing my students to the lions' when they graduate, knowing the problems related to the nursing shortage and the lack of seasoned nurses to mentor the 'young' in the clinical settings."

The sense of overwork is compounded by the faculty shortage. One educator deemed the situation as one of "crisis management! We have major issues with filling faculty positions. In addition, the aging of our faculty causes illness absences for themselves and because of family illnesses. We are scrambling to cover our responsibilities." One simply summed up the challenges she faced in nursing education as "keeping up, and being engaged and passionate when I am dog-dead tired."

We also recognize that educators struggle to stay current in nursing research and clinical practice. As one faculty member put it, it is hard to discern what to teach, "what is nice to know as opposed to what is needed. There has been an explosion of information and development and less time to discuss it." We heard from many nurse educators that one of the stiffest challenges they face is how to convey a vast, ever-increasing universe of nursing knowledge (Diekelmann & Smythe, 2004; Ironside, 2004; Tanner, 1998). One nurse educator responding to the Carnegie-NLN survey said, "The constant change challenges us to keep current not only in teaching but practice itself, especially with all the new technology. Being in clinical practice while teaching helps, though, with this, and I think practicing also actually helps students respect you as you are in the trenches with them." Another respondent explained, "I work and I read, talk with other practicing nurses, but there is always something I haven't had experience with!" Another succinctly summarized the problem all nursing faculty face with finding the most up-to-date practices and information: "Often the new evidence in practice is not in the text."

In every school we visited, we found teachers who, in their effort to bring order and organization to a vast amount of information and content overload, resort to cataloguing. In the classroom, for example, the teacher focuses almost exclusively on organ systems or their diseases, starting with a broad category such as the liver or nutrition, and then introducing sub-categories with their sub-subcategories and their sub-sub-subcategories. The class opens with a brief review of the subject as a whole. The teacher might start with pictures of anatomy, move to some basic physiology, and continue with a list of all the parts of the body and signs of pathology a nurse would need to be aware of in assessment. From assessment, the next topic might be nursing diagnoses for patients, how to implement orders for interventions for patients, and special situations that arise in practice, such as nursing orders for patients with feeding tubes. We observed many classes in which all the information was organized around the nursing process: assessment, analysis and diagnosis, planning, implementation, and evaluation.

"Subsuming things under categories," wrote Logstrup in 1995, "is not the same as productive thinking" (p. 150), and nursing students in these classrooms have few opportunities for developing the productive thinking necessary in nursing practice. Presenting ordered and classified information does little to prepare students to *use* knowledge. The categories, which are classifications or labels, do not give the students any heuristic or imaginative access to the use and relevance of the knowledge in practice situations. Because such frameworks are so abstract, the students struggle to grasp the relevance of all the parts of the catalogue and how the categories are relevant for understanding practical clinical situations.

Moreover, the categories are dim representations of the issues the students will see in practice: patients (especially older patients) seldom have only one category of disease or clinical problem, but they have a complement of social and interpersonal concerns as well. It is impossible for the students to gain a deep and nuanced understanding of the interrelationships of diseases from categories that are flat representations of diagnoses, signs and symptoms of one disease. The diagnoses, signs, and symptoms of a disease are often presented as abstract categories and students find it hard to imagine how these abstractions might guide what they would do in practice.

In the nursing classroom, we often found the teacher posed questions in a call-and-response format, where the answer is known and factual. The teacher was clearly listening for one answer and moved on as soon as she heard it. The students did not appear to need to listen to each other, except to decide whether to hazard a guess. We observed students trying to bring in context, often a brief story about friends or relatives who had trouble with disease or illness. The teacher listened politely, made a comment or two, and turned back to the slides and thus the opportunity for engaging students in a discussion of clinical or related experiences was lost.

Some teachers recognize the flaws of their approach. Commented one, "We can teach in this program, we can teach in that program, and I don't necessarily feel that that's true education, when you become so multitask, that you put everything on a PowerPoint and you pull it out of a drawer." Her colleague added, "*Homogenized* is what I call it."

It was disheartening to hear a nursing educator describe struggling to fit in standardized lectures using PowerPoint slides: "I'm not so accustomed to...[such] structure in the classroom. For example, postpartum has something like 117 slides and the antepartum has 170. I'm more accustomed to not having so many slides and so many PowerPoint presentation handouts and instead presenting an idea and then having case studies and discussion in class and things like that. So it's taking me a while to make sure that I get to other slides. . . . I'm almost afraid I'm the one that colors outside the lines here."

We understand how nursing education could come to this point. On entering academia from hospital training schools (primarily in the early 1960s), nurse educators felt pressured to conform to academia's style of presenting abstract, decontexualized, formal theories. For example, in the late seventies and early eighties, NLN's accreditation criteria required one unifying theoretical framework for every nursing curriculum (Meleis,

2006). This presented many practical problems for a practice as broad and complex as nursing. No one theory could adequately fit the criteria of forming a framework for the whole curriculum. Some theories were too focused on acute care, illness, and injury, while others were too focused on community health, health promotion, and human development. Over the years, NLN dropped this accreditation criterion of a unifying, integrative use of *one* nursing theory (Meleis, 2006); however, it seems that excessive use of taxonomies, as a way of cataloguing information, replaced the quest for formal theoretical frameworks.

The newer taxonomic catalogues fit the notions and classificatory demands of nursing informatics. Bowker and Star (1999) cite the standardization, the clearance of past theories and knowledge as part of the motivation for creating an informatics nomenclature and classification of nursing work from the ground up. The drive for standardization of nursing language was in large measure a strategy for making nursing work more visible, explicit, and retrievable in the health care records (Bowker & Star, 1999).

Influenced by computerized databases and information, the task of the nursing faculty can come to be putting multiple frameworks for classifying and categorizing information on a series of PowerPoint slides. Of course, such a collection of classifications can in no way capture the complexity of the knowledge or the complexity of using knowledge in particular situations.

Thus nurse educators have been encouraged to literally teach North American Nursing Diagnosis Association-International (NANDA-I) Taxonomy of Nursing Diagnoses, Interventions, and Outcomes as the basic scaffolding for classroom teaching. This is the equivalent of using Psychiatric Diagnostic Classifications (DSM IV), which are rarely nonoverlapping, as the primary means for meeting and conducting therapy with particular patients in psychotherapy. In nursing and psychiatry, the taxonomy may be useful in retrieving records, receiving reimbursement, and understanding broad categories of mental illnesses, but the DSM IV does not replicate the thinking process, nor the actual practice of doing psychotherapy, and therefore is a poor portal for teaching the actual habits, skills, and practices of psychotherapy with particular patients with a unique illness history, pattern, and overlapping of symptoms and diseases.

The educational mistake we see playing out in the nursing school classrooms replicates the error of trying to force nursing knowledge and curriculum into *one* theoretical framework for nursing. In this case, it is not a theory that is concretized and reified across all nursing practice contexts, but a much more reduced, structured formal system designed to function within a formal informatics system. This does not help students imagine how they will take up and use relevant knowledge in caring for particular patients with a range of diseases and illness concerns.

Standardization of Lectures

The development of automated presentation software has given teachers the power to standardize lectures, which seemed to be a way to solve the problems of faculty shortage and high turnover rate. In some programs, standardization of lecture meant that any teacher could teach any class; this would, on the surface, seem a boon to a personnel-strapped program. The most extreme case we saw is one school that seeks to standardize the course material across programs, regardless of the individual teacher's interests in or qualifications to teach the classes. Standardization often came in response to trying to enlarge a program through enrolling multiple cohorts of students within the calendar year.

The standardized lecture focuses on information transfer rather than helping students learn what is salient in particular professional practice situations. One group of teachers voiced deep doubts about the use standardized lectures, speaking of the pressure of being "pushed into a little bit of a canned performance, you know. I've probably been the last one to come on board with all the PowerPoint stuff, in our course anyway, and that's been a challenge and it's been sometimes difficult for me. Where I see things, I want to do this in a different order, I want to change this up, I want to teach it a little differently and then sometimes I've been criticized for that." Another teacher said, "And now that's more standardized and so you're kind of having to fit into a mold a little bit more and that's been something I have had a little resistance to. I think in some ways it kind of cramps your style a little bit. You're having to do things according to somebody else's agenda, use a program that somebody else prepared, give a test that you had very little input into."

The packaged lecture can also be used to compensate for a lack of current knowledge. One educator worried about her school, where "none of the faculty teaching the major nursing theory/clinical major courses teach clinical and all are out of step with current clinical practice." With a shortage of nursing faculty and the pressure on programs to serve more students, we fear even more widespread use of this practice. It was not unusual to observe teachers who focus entirely on content and do not spend time in class finding out whether their students understand the material. Generally, these "shows" do not offer access to the knowledge, although course coordinators or educators might assume that they do. Convenience has trumped exploration and curiosity and bewilderingly contradicted or ignored the rich experience that students have in the clinical setting. As one student summed it up, "Across the board, good or bad teachers, there's way too much PowerPoint, way too much PowerPoint."

Team Teaching in the Classroom

Another trend we observed is where several teachers are responsible for teaching one class, or what teachers dubbed team teaching. The use of PowerPoint slides may have made it seem easier for teachers to standardize lectures and team-teach in the classroom. In theory they could share their lectures with one another before they give them and e-mail their slides to each other. In every school we visited, we found team teaching in the classroom or the development of a course by a team of teachers. By *team teaching* we mean courses taught by more than one teacher, with most of the teachers being nurses. There were instances of interdisciplinary team teaching, where a teacher on the team did not have a degree in nursing, and we will return to this idea in later sections, but for the most part the team consisted of nurse educators. Team teaching raises several questions. In the previous section we heard from a teacher who felt disconcerted by not being able to step away from PowerPoint slides. Her course was team-taught, and once it had been developed, each teacher had to teach according to the course program. The teacher told us that she liked her colleagues very much: "We may not be able to change too many things but we at least listen to one another and we definitely back each other up in front of the students." This teacher reported that she and her colleagues had some regular meetings about once a month, but "more often they're just informal little 'grab a half an hour here, do something there.'"

Whether through informal meetings or anecdotal notes, teachers valued communicating with each other, so that students did not fall behind. These meetings, whether informal as they were in some schools or formal standing meetings with planned agendas, were important for faculty as well. One teacher told us about the formal meetings her school hosted, where there was an expectation that the team of teachers would discuss students and support any faculty who had students who were not doing well, as was "J.'s" experience when "six of her ten students were failing in lecture. And so we needed to be supportive of J., who was working so hard in clinical."

Another benefit of team teaching was the different perspectives that each teacher brings to the course material, or as one noted:

> One of the nice things is Nola's a physiologist, I'm a psychologist, and we teach class together. When we first started teaching we would sort of say, "Oh Nola needs to answer that question, she's the physiologist." But, you know, over the years what we've gotten to do is having to work together and learning—getting to know each other and our beliefs and our systems and how my stuff folds in with hers and hers folds in with mine. I think what we have to offer the students is both perspectives.

Faculty who team-taught, though, did not always agree on how to approach the material they taught. One noted about her team teaching: "My colleague believes that everyone should understand data at a higher level. I have a tendency to bring it down some because I know that there are those students who maybe don't have a strong science background and are struggling."

Some faculty identified other problems of consistency or not knowing what their colleagues were doing. As one put it: "We have this idea that these words were said in class, therefore the students have learned the content. Well no, they haven't. One of the problems we face is that we have people coming and going, so we have people who don't know what's being taught."

Although they worried about coordinating their work adequately, which may explain the many references we heard to informal conversation in the hallway or a shared office, with few exceptions faculty members reported that their team teaching or co-teaching went well. Teachers indicated that they talked with each other about students and the teaching as they went along. Teachers seemed to find their conversation with colleagues helped them teach better, which raises a question we will return to in the conclusion about how to create opportunities for teachers to meet and discuss teaching.

Given that many nurse educators found team teaching to be positive and given the pressures they face in keeping up to date in practice, not to mention new scholarship from the humanities and the natural and social sciences, we are puzzled that more schools did not have teams of nurses teach with teachers from other fields. We understand the high value nurse educators and students place on nurses teaching nursing students and the need for domain-specific teaching, but faculty report overwhelmingly that they are overloaded. Many also reported they were asked to teach in areas they did not know well or had not kept up to date. Teachers from other fields might be able to relieve some of this pressure, if they received adequate preparation on how to weave their knowledge in the humanities and natural and social sciences into the domain-specific teaching of nurse educators.

Teaching and Learning in the Classroom and Skills Laboratories

Students recognize that naming and categorizing yields a low level of understanding, with little connection to practice. One student described her classes as "taught in an old-fashioned science curriculum sort of way, when a different approach may be more suited." As students noted, with such an approach it is all too easy for a teacher to move through a lecture at a fast clip, reading the slides. As one student noted, "I think it keeps them on task. They have a certain curriculum they need to cover and it's their way of guaranteeing to themselves that these things did get covered. And also it helps sort of take the responsibility off them as far as making sure the material got out there to students. . . . And so, I think it's easier for the instructor but not necessarily better for the student. I think [PowerPoint] is a good tool, but I don't like the way that instructors rely on it so much."

One student described a lecture as "a very prescribed, static environment that moves at a certain pace and there's no room to stop if a quarter of the class isn't following. It's not an interactive environment. And it just doesn't sit well with me as far as, you know, what I know about educating others and my own excitement about learning." Students appreciate when teachers resist the canned lecture. One student described with admiration a faculty member in her pathophysiology class who "was able to step away from the PowerPoint format and realize . . . especially with electrolyte balance, a good half of us were just not on board. We didn't have the science. So she took it back a notch and she explained that. I still didn't get it, but at least she explained it to me."

Another student pinpointed a variety of issues in the classroom:

> Well, can I say what doesn't make a fantastic teacher? Maybe we can work from there. I think that PowerPoint is the bane of my school's existence and what some instructors have now decided to do is to go through the book, maybe even the night before, and make slides from the book and then stand up in front of class with their PowerPoint slides and proceed to read to us directly, the entire lecture, what is written on their slides, including maybe poor grammar or misspellings

that are on the slides, will come out verbatim. And if you were to ask any questions about maybe what a word actually meant on the slide, they don't actually know. They just typed it because they copied it out of the book. And that is so disappointing. Now, not every instructor in this program does that, certainly, but to have that type of instruction in an institution like this was hugely disappointing. And there is this huge shortage of nursing instructors and as a result, I think some people have gotten pulled into nursing instruction.... Teaching is an art. It's not just something that anybody can do. And so they were nurses, not teachers. But then they've been in this role now for, what, seven, eight years and now they've lost kind of contact with, like as technology has changed with the nursing portion of it and now they're not even that good as nurses. So now we don't have either. We don't really have a really good nurse and we don't have a really good teacher. We have something mediocre, something in the middle, and that's frustrating.

Most distressingly, students wonder whether their teachers are using appropriate approaches. In general, students reported that their classroom teachers lecture without examples of what they might see in clinical settings. As one student said, "The instructors do not give enough clinical examples of how the material relates to what we need to know as nurses."

Games and Entertainment in the Classroom

We observed that the focus on lecture has another side: the need to engage students as much as possible. As one teacher noted:

When you're teaching, you're basically giving a performance, and I view it as that because you have to be able to keep the students engaged, and particularly this generation. You know, they're used to sound bites and quick e-mails and instant messaging. I try to stay as relevant as I possibly can to what's happening in their world and their generation but also what's happening in the world and to make the class—I hate to even call it "lecture"...I truly believe that if they're not engaged and interactive and interested then they're not going to be understanding the material. I also want them to be excited about what they're learning, beyond taking the exam, you know, into graduation, beyond graduation.

This teacher's goal is admirable, and one that we heard echoed by many teachers.

To engage their students, some teachers made good use of humor in their classes. For example, teachers told stories with a gentle humor about their nursing experience or about relatives or friends to illustrate a clinical point. Other teachers used games to present opportunities for students to interact with each other. For example, to teach gastrointestinal anatomy, one educator gave each student a card naming a section of the gut; the students had to organize themselves in a line, in the order that food would pass through the system. Following the order of the cards, the teacher discussed specific diseases and problems, such as gastrointestinal obstruction. One purpose of the activity, the teacher explained, was to invite the students to solve problems together, and the teacher found that the activity brought "them into lecture with more energy than they normally have." In fact, this game was quite effective in actively engaging the students in relevant learning about the anatomy and pathophysiology of the gastrointestinal tract. It was more than a mere guessing game.

Although the students' attention is gained through games, the quality of their attentiveness may fall short of serious engagement with the practice of nursing. Whether the teacher intends it or not, games can reinforce the idea that guessing is acceptable and that memorization is the major learning goal in nursing education. From the teacher's use of games in the classroom, students may infer a subtle message that the intellectual projects and caregiving issues of nursing practice are not appealing enough to draw students' attention.

Games and entertainment sometimes had unintended consequences. At their worst, we found practices designed to enliven the material that in reality trivialized course material or encouraged students to guess. One teacher asks her students to make presentations on a topic and then devise a game to assess learning in the class. She describes it: "Everybody got an answer. They drew out of a bag and they all had an answer and then the person who was presenting said, 'OK, now, for 500 points, this is a test question and one of you has the answer. Who has the answer?' And so he would read the question and then everybody sat there looking at each other. 'Oh, I have it!' But it was fun. So that's how they must assess learning, by creating a game." The teacher felt that "the fun part" for her was to watch the students develop the games. In terms of assessment, students were asked not to generate correct answers but to see whether they had the correct answer, which seems to us to trivialize the complex information that nurses need to know in the clinical setting.

In the most extreme example of entertainment we witnessed, the teacher set up an elaborate game modeled after a television game show. Over the three-hour class period, the teacher offered handmade "prizes," including a cardboard color television for which the students competed. One of her students expressed appreciation for her efforts, explaining that she did not need to take notes or even pay attention. One noted that the game reviewed material they had already covered, and "since it a lot of it was review information and a lot of it we did have basic knowledge on, we could apply our basic knowledge to the games, the game setting. But if it was information that we knew nothing on, that was totally new, then we would probably maybe feel a little bit differently."

Another form of entertainment entails a teacher imitating patient symptoms. It is tricky for the teacher to find the right tone, as we found at one school. A student told us about one performance, adding the comment: "Now, everybody's going to have to admit, that was probably one of our most fun days of class." He explained that the teacher took a break and returned to class as a bipolar patient in the midst of a manic episode and acted the part for forty-five minutes. The student laughed throughout his account of the class: "I'll [laughter] I'll never forget bipolar. I had patients with bipolar in the unit, but always, that'll probably be in mind. I was laughing at home from the [performance], at home, five hours after it happened, and I, you know, I even sent her an e-mail. I said, 'I'm still laughing.' [laughter] You know because it was so, much of it was fun, but yet you would learn, I mean, you learned a lot, from that."

The teacher admitted that she had reservations about how students might interpret her performance:

> And then sometimes I like to just do something way off the wall, and I think when I describe one of my—I don't know if it's best practice of teaching but it's certainly one that gets the students' attention, and I get a lot of positive feedback from and that is when we talk about our mood disorders. I tell them I have a guest speaker to come in and talk to them about mania. I leave the room and I come back quite manic, dressed up, lots of makeup on and for an hour I teach the rest of the class, pacing the class, inappropriately taking their purses and putting them over my shoulder, and walking around, just things that would be typical for someone who was in a manic phase. So then I ask them, "What are you going to do for me? What are you going to do for me?" and I get them to tell me what interventions are needed and we talk about the medications, and I also make sure that I always tell them that . . . because they're laughing the whole time. I know this is funny, that it's totally unexpected from me, but I don't want them to misunderstand that I think this illness is at all funny. Part of what I

want them to see is what it's like to be with someone for an hour who just won't stop moving or talking and getting in their faces and moving around, but that it's not an effort to make fun of someone who has quite a crippling illness. So they really seem to like that and it always show up on my faculty evaluation. I don't know what other people outside of my class might think of that. I don't know what word to use but "display," maybe.

The teacher was concerned about how her performance would be taken, and she wondered how her students interpreted it. She was aware that her students liked the act and seemed glad that they commented favorably on it in her faculty evaluations. Her students said that the value lay in the teacher using the performance as part of a scenario and asking them throughout about interventions and medications. The students, however, did report that they were still laughing hours later. We think the teacher's reflection signals that she is struggling with a sense that she also needs to convey the human side of the illness and find a way for students to better understand the difficulties persons with bipolar disease have in managing their illness. From her students' reports, it sounds as if she might emphasize more the human suffering of bipolar disease, for example, by including a more rounded portrayal of this devastating illness.

The use of games raises another set of questions. A number of students mentioned that they appreciate the classroom as theater, where educators might make jokes or, as one teacher did, lie on the ground suddenly and ask, "Now what do you do?" We found that student evaluations of faculty, which students in most schools complete at the end of each course, play a decisive role in faculty decisions about how to structure their classes, as the faculty member who pretended to be bipolar mentioned in her interview. At several schools, student evaluations are taken for granted as accurate assessments of teaching, or so we can hear from this dean: "I've been a teacher twenty-eight years and I've been a department chair, so I've seen a lot of student evaluations for different faculty, and in general, they're pretty on the mark." She went on to say that they "are consistent with the reality." This administrator felt that student evaluations of teaching were consistently reliable and valid. However, we note that what students like in a class may not be what they need, as we heard from the students who enjoyed the faculty member imitating a bipolar patient. Faculty evaluations may not be a good indicator of the quality of student learning. It can be difficult for students to pinpoint what they need, in part because they may not know what they are missing.

One teacher we interviewed illustrated this in her appraisal of a class that she took over from her colleagues. Reflecting on what the course was accomplishing, she removed a game modeled on the television game show *Jeopardy*. In her opinion, there was too much class time devoted to games, and too little to learning. She noted:

> I did make major changes. . . .. They were using two or three of the twelve weeks to play a Jeopardy game, which was student interaction, question/answer, and that particular format, and I went back to a traditional lecture format. Our pharmacology sections of the boards. . .were starting to decline in pharmacology, so frankly I was trying to look at some other methods to help them retain information. Also, I don't know how to play Jeopardy, frankly.

The paradigm educators whose teaching we describe in Parts Two, Three, and Four do not use games. They elicit student engagement by giving the students intellectual and moral challenges of reasoning about real patient situations. They involve the students in exercising a sense of salience, in developing clinical imagination, and exploring ethical comportment. They understand that every aspect of the education experience, whether in clinical settings or the classroom, conveys messages that the students interpret to be about the profession and that therefore affect the students' formation as nurses.

Skills Laboratories

We had the opportunity to observe many classes and their associated skills laboratory. For example, we observed a conscientious teacher give a thorough and well-organized lecture on the care of patients with nutrition, hydration, and elimination needs. Then we watched as students were taught in their skills laboratory the basic skills for taking care of such patients. The students appeared to attach more importance to some of the skills than others. For example, they were far more engaged with and concerned about the technology of the intravenous machine than about the intricacies they might encounter in positioning a patient with a fractured hip who needs to use a bedpan. Perhaps the machine seemed emblematic of the type of practitioner they wanted to be, one well versed in the complex technology of care, not someone who does everyday hygiene or body care. They recognize that they will certainly need to know the ins and outs of intravenous machines. The machines were new to them, high-tech and high-status, while taking care of patients with elimination problems can be slightly embarrassing for the novice and seem less important. But how nursing students comport themselves in the poorly veiled private spaces created by thin curtains around a bed represents a major lesson in professionalization. Students must learn to balance an immobilized patient's need for privacy, where safety, comfort, and hygiene must be taken into account, with the challenge of how to safely move the patient on and off a small plastic bedpan. When nursing faculty enter their classroom, many seem to leave behind this complex world of practice, where students must learn equally well the lessons of all three apprenticeships that are needed to insert a needle into a patient's vein to deliver fluid by means of a complex machine that in a few hours they will remove in a plastic pan.

Fragmentation

Nursing education is fragmented. Teams of teachers teach different parts of courses; depending on the team, they might compare their teaching in brief hallway chats. Clinical, skills laboratory, and classroom are separated, often with instructors for each one.

To compound the problem, we found that the classroom-clinical divide exacerbates the fragmentation that students feel. The nursing curriculum leaves students to their own devices to piece together what they learn from a number of courses. As one student said of her curriculum, "Sometimes it seems we are in a correspondence course. We have to get it on our own." Another student offered, "I think it would be helpful to have more integration of the content of our courses. I understand you can't have one big course, or maybe you could, but in our nursing process type class they say they don't cover meds because they say you'll get that in pharmacology and pathophysiology. And I think it would it would be nice to have it come together in [a] big piece, the whole picture, instead of having to go through and kind of match things up."

To be sure, some faculty try to integrate clinical and classroom learning, but students note that their experience can vary widely. One student observed, "Some students are lucky enough to obtain a clinical instructor that also teaches the course. Then the course objectives and content are better facilitated with direct clinical setting examples. An example might be an instructor teaching, 'Remember, we talked about this subject in class ... here is a prime example of that lecture in the clinical setting.' Pointing out real examples solidifies classroom taught information."

The phrase "lucky enough" underscores the opposite experience of many students. In many programs, clinical and classroom instruction is not formally coordinated so that instructors could cross-reference topics and experiences from one to the other. Moreover, many students are not lucky enough to have a classroom teacher who brings in the students' immediate experiences of patients and families, or who anticipates examples of what the students might see in a clinical setting, either from habit of teaching style or lack of current experience. As one student acknowledged, it can be hard for faculty to make these connections: "My program tries to incorporate our clinical experiences with the classroom content as much as possible. It is difficult, however, to predict what disease processes will be present on your clinical day to correlate to lecture content, and I think that they do the best that they can."

Such fragmentation contributes to a sense of overload. Nursing students universally complain about lack of time for sleep, completion of assignments, and learning what they need to master for nursing practice. One refrain was "so much to learn in such a short time." Students astutely pointed to what one called "unnecessary busy work that is not relevant to current nursing practice." Another student observed, "There is no time to actually learn the material. I feel like I'm running through a maze to get everything read and done, but no time to actually learn it." In site visits and responses to the surveys conducted in collaboration with the NLN and AACN, educators also referred to fragmentation. One faculty member observed, "It is almost like the material in each course is learned for that course, then boxed up and put on a shelf somewhere in their brain."

Toward a Goal of Integration

More than one student suggested, "There have to be other ways." Taking the students' call for a more effective approach a step further, we believe that nursing students need to learn for a practice, and every class should contribute to their clinical imagination. In this chapter we describe the struggle of many classroom teachers to "cover" content using taxonomies of diseases or nursing diagnosis. These taxonomies can lead to academic overload or, as students called it, too much busy work.

The busy work and overload came about, in part, from the move nursing educators made when they transferred nursing education to academic settings. In these new settings, they encountered pressure to increase the prestige of nursing education. In response, they emulated other fields that valued abstract, formal, and classificatory knowledge. Coping with the pressures to increase nursing's prestige and the explosion of nursing and medical knowledge have led to an encyclopedic approach to teaching in the classroom.

The nursing classroom in particular needs to be a place of rich and powerful learning, and much of this book addresses this issue and offers examples of effective classroom teaching. Nursing educators must teach for a practice that works deliberately in the in-between social spaces of mechanistic medical diagnosis and treatment and the patients' lived experience of illness or prevention of illness in their particular life, family, and community. They must help their students gain solid theoretical and practical bases in psychology, anthropology, and sociology as well as in the humanities. Yet we found high variability in both the quality and depth of teaching and learning in the humanities and natural and social sciences, all of which are necessary for nursing.

We recognize the tremendous pressure that nurse educators are under to "deliver" an exponentially increasing body of information. Finding a more effective approach to teaching the knowledge base and helping students learn to use that knowledge effectively in their practice and ethical comportment is one of nursing education's great challenges. It is best achieved through integrating all three professional apprenticeships, the knowledge base, skilled know-how, and clinical reasoning and ethical comportment, in all teaching and learning settings. When nursing educators help students integrate what they learn in the three apprenticeships, rather than when they separate them, students develop a moral sense of what it is good to be and do in a situation, on the basis of knowledge and research, as well as learning skilled know-how (Benner, 1984; Benner & Wrubel, 1982; Benner et al., 2009; Benner et al., 1999).

To bring about the important changes nursing education requires, educators must address their own practice-education gap and learn new ways to approach the practice of teaching, especially in the classroom. In the course of our study, we were inspired by nursing educators who are meeting the challenges with creativity. We observed many examples of innovative nurse educators who are at once faithful to nursing's historic commitment to patient care yet also teaching the depth and breadth of knowledge needed by today's nurses.

Taking the students' call, we offer in the next chapter different and more effective ways to change thinking about and approaches to nursing education.

4

A NEW APPROACH TO NURSING EDUCATION

BECAUSE NURSING PRACTICE demands both depth and breadth of knowledge in many areas, the problem of asking students to learn a great deal in a brief period cannot easily be resolved.

It is tempting to allow the current crises of the nursing shortage to distract from the need to make important changes in nursing education to increase the quality of prelicensure education. Yet the practice-education gap, the undereducation of nurses in prelicensure programs, and insufficient continuing nursing education for those in practice are, we believe, at least as serious a set of problems as the shortage of nurses and nurse educators. The nursing shortage must be addressed through changes in both structure and approach to teaching and learning.

As we mentioned in the previous chapters, we believe that nursing education must commit to important structural changes. These include requiring the baccalaureate as the entrance to practice, introducing nursing courses in the first year of the baccalaureate program, increasing second-degree baccalaureate and master's programs, improving students' efficient progress from ADN programs to baccalaureate and master's programs, requiring a postgraduate year of internship in a clinical setting, and more.

We know that making such structural changes will require considerable time and funding. Moreover, these needed structural reforms—extensions of the period of formal education for nurses—are only part of the answer. The time in nursing school must be used more effectively. As the previous chapters describing teaching in the clinical setting and the classroom suggest, nursing education has considerable strengths, especially experiential learning, along with effective pedagogies such as coaching. Nursing education must bring these effective teaching strategies into the classroom. Moreover, the educational experience must model and promote integration across the professional apprenticeships: knowledge, skilled know-how, and ethical comportment. Toward these ends, we offer a new way of thinking about nursing education.

Many nurse educators tend to valorize a narrow form of reasoning, trying to teach students to stand outside a given situation to take a snapshot view of it and make a rational choice about an action. Perhaps in an effort to follow an "academic" approach, some nurse educators try to teach students to interpret a situation with formal, unchanging, or standardized criteria based on abstract properties and directives that come from outside the situation. In effect, this suggests to the student that any situation can be made completely explicit and that different situations can be made comparable by using generalized assumptions and formal criteria for making judgments. This approach works only up to a point, where the decision maker can verify that all the assumptions made about the situation are precisely the same and that the criteria are appropriate (Taylor, 1993). However, in evolving situations that are underdetermined, that cannot be made completely explicit, which is the norm in today's nursing practice, the nurse must take into account patient trends over time. The critical pathways guidelines or formal decision-making strategies do not fit every situation, and it is misleading to suggest that these are anything but guides. Again, approaching nursing education through domain-specific teaching brings a more effective focus to teaching clinical reasoning across patient transitions (a form of practical reasoning).

Four Essential Shifts for Integration

Nursing educators must strive for deeper, more effective integration of the three professional apprenticeships. To that end, we suggest that teachers change their assumptions about teaching and their approach to fostering student learning in four ways, two of which we review briefly here because we have already discussed them in Chapters Two and Three. We describe the second two shifts more extensively because they are being introduced in this chapter.

We suggest that nurse educators:

1. *Shift from a focus on covering decontextualized knowledge to an emphasis on teaching for a sense of salience, situated cognition, and action in particular situations.*

As we noted in Chapter Three, many teachers organize their classes around lists of abstract taxonomies, or other abstract theory and knowledge, which gives their students little or no indication about how to integrate the knowledge they present in a practice context. We found most troubling the ubiquity of the strategy of presenting theories and clinical knowledge as taxonomic naming systems. Few students can imagine how the classification systems can be used in their actual direct patient care. Although learning classification systems is integral to mastering and retrieving information systems (Bowker & Star, 1999), these systems are not sufficient. Instead of presenting flat representations of multiple taxonomic structures, or "cataloguing," nursing educators need to help students learn to use nursing knowledge and science. For example, teachers might develop computer-based exercises as part of learning various nursing documentation and care-planning strategies. Students can also learn taxonomies in the context of critiquing, updating, and improving practice in a particular situation.

Precious classroom time could then be used instead for developing a sense of salience about what is important and unimportant about a clinical situation. As Bourdieu (1990) points out, the heart of practical reasoning requires understanding the nature of the situation. Nurses work in complex, relatively unstructured clinical situations where they must learn to quickly recognize and assess what is most and least important. Because practice situations are underdetermined, are open-ended, and change over time, practitioners must first grasp the nature of the situation before they can act intelligently and prudently. It is not possible for the student to build up a holistic grasp of the situation element by element in an actual complex practice situation. The most that can be arranged or controlled is for the instructor to assign the student patients who are not in crisis and who require relatively simple, straightforward interventions. Continued situated coaching is required for the student to grasp the changing relevance, and demands, resources, and constraints in a particular situation, and therefore it entails developing a sense of salience, what Eraut (1994) calls a productive form of knowledge *use* and Lave and Wenger (1991) call situated cognition. Over time, students effectively shift to what they can *notice* (drawing on their background understanding) in the situation without deliberate prompting and place their focused attention (put in the foreground) on more novel aspects of the situation. Developing a sense of salience requires linking perception and discernment with the ability to use knowledge from a rich knowledge base.

2. *Shift from a sharp separation of clinical and classroom teaching to integration of classroom and clinical teaching.*

As we discuss in Chapters Two and Three, we observed in all schools of nursing a sharp divide between classroom and clinical teaching, and the students notice the significant difference between their experiences in both. A formal separation of clinical and classroom teaching does not support a complex, integrated use of knowledge and skills that nursing practice demands.

Unfortunately, we observed many situations where teachers expect students to perform, demonstrate, or present a given skill out of clinical context, usually in a skills laboratory. It can be helpful to use a nonclinical setting to teach first-year nursing students how to take vital signs or other elemental competencies. If teachers present only simple, stripped-down examples or test students on elemental competencies, they may not help students prepare for many clinical situations. To take a common example, when students learn to measure blood pressure, they often learn in simplified and decontextualized situations where they are taking blood pressure measurements on healthy individuals. These tasks are fine as a starting point. But they do not prepare a student to make a clinical assessment about, for example, a hypertensive patient in labor and delivery, where the student must move quickly in interpreting information from the patient's vital signs and taking account of the particulars in the situation. Lists of broad areas of competent performance, such as those enumerated by the Institute of Medicine and used in the Quality and Safety in Nursing Education project (Cronenwett et al., 2007), demonstrate an integrative view of clinical performance rather than emphasize narrowly prescribed lists of elemental competencies. By integrating clinical and classroom learning into a seamless whole, nurse educators could address the fragmentation students currently experience and take some of the burden of overload off themselves, their colleagues, and the students.

3. *Shift from an emphasis on critical thinking to an emphasis on clinical reasoning and multiple ways of thinking that include critical thinking.*

Explicit respect for practical reasoning and multiple ways of thinking is needed. Such respect would allow nursing education to reformulate the role of critical thinking. Nursing education has fallen into the habit of using "critical thinking" as a catch-all phrase for the many forms of thinking that nurses use in practice—an unfortunate misnomer. Students need to learn which situations require critical thinking and which do not. Thus students use critical reflection when they pose questions about an event, patient, or situation that can help draw their attention to a new interpretation. For example, students use critical reflection when they deconstruct situations of practice breakdown, or failure of outmoded theories; they also use it when they question received ideas and practices that need reform or innovation. Yet critical reflection cannot be the only focus, or even the primary one, in learning any professional practice. Nurses need multiple ways of thinking, such as clinical reasoning and clinical imagination as well as critical, creative, scientific, and formal criterial reasoning. By clinical reasoning, we mean the ability to reason as a clinical situation changes, taking into account the context and concerns of the patient and family. When nurses use clinical reasoning, they capture patients' trends and trajectories. Nurses use a related way of thinking about patients when they use clinical imagination to conjure up possibilities, resources, and constraints in the patient and family situations. Nurse educators develop their students' clinical imagination and reasoning by asking what-if questions about a patient or the family (what if a blood test or other laboratory test changes?). All nurses also use critical, creative, scientific, and formal criterial reasoning. Like physicians, lawyers, and engineers, nurses are expected to keep their practice up to date, using their clinical judgment to discern when a body of published research is relevant for a particular patient and how sound and well established the scientific base is. For example, confronting a patient with acute respiratory distress, low blood pressure, and an extremely slow pulse, the nurse must take quick action from a well-established scientific understanding of the functioning of the lungs, the direction of the circulatory system, causes for slow heart rate, low blood pressure, and so on. When quick action and therapeutic interventions are required, evidence-based knowledge, the accepted standards of practice, and good clinical reasoning are essential.

Classroom teachers often give students models of how they should think about problems, such as models of critical thinking. They describe these decontextualized and mentalistic representations of critical thinking or the nursing problem-solving process as "frameworks of thinking." A framework of thinking, however, is not the same as thinking. This problem is not unique to nursing education. Sullivan and Rosin (2008) note that the critical thinking agenda in higher education seeks to help students disengage from context-bound, concrete knowledge to what is considered a "higher" form of knowledge made explicit, formal, operational, and more abstract and general. They state: "Virtually all educational programs to develop critical thinking imagine their aim as teaching students to abstract general rules from specific contexts and thereby to inculcate the priority of analytical over concrete or intuitive thinking. This agenda overlooks the embodied, often tacit knowledge present in skillful judgment. Knowledge is reduced exclusively to formal or representational modes" (pp. 99–100).

Thinking like a nurse requires clinical reasoning, as well as critical, creative, scientific, and formal criterial reasoning. Cynicism and excessive doubt, often the by-product of *overuse* of reflective critical thinking, will not help the nurse draw on appropriate knowledge and act in a particular situation. Nor does critical thinking *alone* develop students' perceptual acuity or clinical imagination about using science, skilled know-how, and practical knowledge in a particular situation. Clinical imagination is required for students to grasp the nature of patients' needs as they change over time. Likewise, narrative understanding and interpretation of clinical situations help to enrich the student's clinical imagination and reasoning about changes in the patient's condition over time. Situated learning is also vital. By this we mean students learn by, through, and in situations that involve particular patients, whether the situation involves patients in a clinical setting or in paper cases or simulations. Students must experience practice, or learn experientially, in particular situations. Critical reflection, analysis, and thinking are essential to all education. However, they are most effectively developed when teachers understand their goals and functions in relation to practice.

4. *Shift from an emphasis on socialization and role taking to an emphasis on formation.*

Nursing education engages theories about socialization, roles and role taking, role making, and role performance. Ideas drawn from role theory and socialization (Grusec & Hastings, 2007) are useful in any practice discipline that must coordinate and link role functions with other disciplines and team members. But socialization in any simple view is not the best way to describe formation, those changes in identity and self-understanding that occur in moving from being a lay person to a professional. Formation of student nurses occurs within their skilled practices and highly relational work, literally transforming their ways of perceiving and acting in situations. Formation describes the practitioner's evolving experience from that perspective, while socialization describes the social forces and influences on the person's formative experience. Socialization strategies that influence one practitioner may not be as formative for another. By using the notion of formation, we seek to signal a more constitutive and transactional view of formation within a profession that includes agency, commitments, practice capacities, and identification with the profession's notions of the good as well as standards.

To become a good nurse, one must develop not only technical expertise but also the ability to form helping relationships and engage in practical ethical and clinical reasoning (Dreyfus, Dreyfus, & Benner, 2009). Becoming a nurse is thus best articulated as *formation* because it points to being constituted by the meanings, content, intents, and practice of nursing rather than merely learning or being socialized into a nursing role in an external way. We use the philosophical term *constituted* because it points to a theory of meaning that includes being formed so that one can dwell and act effectively in terms of taken-for-granted self-understandings and meanings, rather than just imitating or mimicking them. This is why we like Margaret Mohrmann's metaphor of dance to describe formation. Especially in nursing and medicine, where ethical formation occurs through learning in situations, the metaphor of dance is more accurate than imagining static shapes or forms that the learner imitates. Formation allows for and can stimulate innovation evident in many forms of dance:

> Formation refers to the method by which a person is prepared for a particular task or is made capable of functioning in a particular role. One forms, as well as educates, priests, soldiers, nurses, and doctors in a process that moves beyond the knowledge content of those crafts to the moral content of the practices—the obligations entailed, the demands imposed—and thus to the moral formation of the practitioners. Moreover, it is generally the case that one is formed toward something, some telos, some ideal shape or condition.... A better metaphor [for being true to form] is dance: having and displaying integrity is more a matter of being able to move in ways that are consistent with the originating and developing themes of our lives. Teachers, guides, and practice make us better dancers because they help us listen more carefully and follow the music we hear more confidently. We learn which movements fit the rhythms and which do not [Mohrmann, 2006, pp. 93–95].

In interviews and survey responses, many nursing students described profound changes in their sense of identity, explaining how the experience of skilled practice and highly relational work transformed the way they perceive and act. Students identified particular learning experiences as affecting their capacity to act in the future, increasing their self-knowledge and understanding, or reassuring them of their chosen profession. They develop moral imagination or the ability to imagine the moral content inherent in the practice of nursing.

As we describe in depth in Part Four, we suggest that nursing educators urge more intentional use of these transformational experiences and emphasize formation of professional identity more than socialization. *Transformation* and *formation*, terms that we borrow from Carnegie's study of clergy education (Foster et al., 2005), address the development of the senses, aesthetics, perceptual acuities, relational skills, knowledge, and dispositions that take place as student nurses form professional identity.

There is another important aspect of formation that we call to nursing educators' attention. Although the process of formation is one of the strengths of U.S. nursing education, it is important for nurse educators to recognize that formation—shaping of the habits and dispositions for use of knowledge and skilled-know-how—occurs in *every* aspect of a nursing student's education. It happens not only when knowledge is acquired, or beliefs are changed, but also in the midst of caring for patients, in engaging in the situated practice of nursing. Teaching that stops short of effective formation at best leaves the learner with only abstract knowledge not yet accessible in practice situations. Formation requires skilled know-how, embodied capacities to act in practice situations when the patient's well-being is at stake. However, students are formed by all they do, all they perceive and interpret, and all models of practice—not only in the context of what they think or know intellectually but also in terms of their skilled capacities, their grasp of the notions of good nursing practice, and their taken-for-granted assumptions and expectations.

In other words, formation occurs through the formal curriculum; in implicit curricular agendas or hidden curriculum; in the formal and informal teaching in the classroom and clinical settings; and in dialogues with patients, other students, nurses, other health care providers, and faculty. Formation occurs during PowerPoint slide presentations and pathophysiology-themed games of Jeopardy or The Million Dollar Question as well as during coaching, feedback sessions, clinical conferences, and the student's own process of reflection. Formation also occurs in the gaps. For example, students notice discrepancies between what is presented in the classroom and what happens in practice. As one student said, in a comment representative of something we heard consistently during our site visits, "The nurses that I work with, I've asked them over and over about nursing process, what the nursing theories and nursing diagnoses are ... it's frustrating, it's a lot of paperwork, and they laugh at me. They say, 'Nobody uses that.'" No assessment of a nursing program or curriculum would thus be complete without consideration of the full import of the students' experience and the understanding of the profession that the students are likely to derive from it. A shift to a student-focused sense of transformation and reflection on formative experiences in nursing school would enrich the student's sense of identity and self-understanding as a nurse.

That formation is, for better or worse, a product of the students' experience suggests that nursing educators consider carefully all aspects of the program, including pedagogies, assessments, and curricula. For example, both students and faculty spoke consistently of moments of transformation that reveal to the student what it is to be a nurse, the moral responsibility of being a nurse. It is impossible to predict what experiences will be pivotal for a student; nor is it possible to quantify how many revelations large and small accumulate, but in the course of our research it became clear that furnishing an experiential learning environment and reflection on that experiential learning across the nursing curriculum supports formation.

In sum, we suggest faculty and students make four shifts in their thinking and approach to nursing education:

1. From a focus on covering decontextualized knowledge to an emphasis on teaching for a sense of salience, situated cognition, and action in particular clinical situations

2. From a sharp separation of classroom and clinical teaching to integrative teaching in all settings

3. From an emphasis on critical thinking to an emphasis on clinical reasoning and multiple ways of thinking that include critical thinking

4. From an emphasis on socialization and role taking to an emphasis on formation

Paradigm Cases of Excellence in Nursing Education

We chose three teachers who have a vision for nursing education's future, and we present them as paradigm cases in Parts Two, Three, and Four. In their teaching, the classroom becomes a place of rich and powerful learning, where students can safely rehearse for complex practice. They take a broader view of rationality in nursing education, whereby students learn multiple ways of thinking and knowledge use, reflect on their practice, engage in clinical inquiry, learn through experience, and articulate their developing experience-based practical knowledge. They stopped teaching a version of clinical reasoning that mimics scientific reasoning. They shifted their emphasis to teaching students how to use knowledge acquired in the classroom in particular clinical situations. They stopped seeing classifications of knowledge, such as those for signs and symptoms, as sufficient unto themselves and instead developed ways of giving students the means to think about the signs and symptoms a particular patient may have, how to interpret them, and what to do about them. In short, in their clinical and classroom teaching these teachers have found ways to engage students in learning in each of the apprenticeships for complex knowledge use and practice. Their teaching strategies are the very ones common to clinical instruction, where educators call on their students to both develop and integrate the three apprenticeships of professional education: knowledge, skilled know-how and clinical reasoning, and ethical formation. We recommend support for teachers to learn to scaffold their courses around patient care. As we illustrate in the paradigm cases, such pedagogies are unfolding case studies, narrative structures for making a case, simulation exercises, and patient interviews. These bring patients into focus to form a basis from which students rehearse aloud, or by in-class writing assignments, the appropriate care of communities, patients, and their families in particular situations.

A paradigm case is defined as a *strong instance* of a pattern or style of performance that embodies skilled know-how and understandings and multiple key meanings of a social practice. The strong instance or paradigm case (Benner, 1994) can be recognized as a pattern of meanings, habits, intents, and styles. Our descriptions of the paradigm-case teachers are based on observations of these teachers in their classrooms and clinical settings. We also interviewed these faculty and a sample of their students outside the classroom, asking them about their understanding of what they were learning in the classroom and clinical settings.

These teachers' teaching and learning practices gave us new insights and suggested a new approach to teaching for the complex practice of nursing. As we considered how each has found ways to solve many difficult discipline-specific pedagogical problems and developed innovative teaching strategies tailored for learning the complex caring practice of nursing, even in environments either unaware of or unsympathetic to their work, we began to articulate the shifts in teaching outlined above. We saw in these teachers new possibilities for nursing education, shifts in approach that would make way for, complement, and enhance the many needed structural changes that nursing education must also effect.

Above all, we chose the three teachers, Diane Pestolesi, Lisa Day, and Sarah Shannon, as paradigm cases because they instantiate the care of the patient in their intents, their concerns, and how they point out salience and meaning in particular clinical situations. They understand that the responsibility of nursing education is equipping students with the necessary cognitive skills and preparing them to act as moral agents—whether they are at the bedside, with a family, or in a community—in situations that are underdetermined, contingent, and changing over time. Thus they make every effort to teach their students how to *be* a nurse in terms of *using* evidenced-based knowledge, clinical judgment, and skilled know-how. Whether in the classroom or the clinical setting, these teachers give their students access to thinking and performing like a nurse in practice.

In each paradigm-case chapter, we augment the paradigm cases with examples drawn from other teachers as well.

Taken together, the paradigm cases illustrate several possible solutions to the challenges and problems we identify in nursing education. Each paradigm case highlights teaching styles that integrate the three apprenticeships of learning in professional education, unify clinical and classroom teaching, and teach from a stance of practice.

PART TWO

TEACHING FOR A SENSE OF SALIENCE

I learn better in a clinical setting. Once I actually do it, I have a better understanding of it, and plus I think that often you have to make a lot of different adjustments for different things, depending on each different patient. You can't really do that in a classroom setting. You can think about what would it be if this patient was this way or that way, but once you actually encounter it, then it sticks with you. You won't forget it.

As THIS STUDENT nurse observes, just as the differences between formal textbook descriptions of signs and symptoms and patients' actual manifestations of illness are great, so is the gap in learning from reading and learning by working in a clinical practice setting (Benner, 2005).

Nursing students must constantly make connections between the physiology and pathophysiology presented in textbooks or classroom lectures and what they find in actual situations with patients. Then they must go a step further and connect that information to implications for assessments and interventions. However, the link between abstract knowledge of physiology and pathophysiology conveyed in the classroom and the implications for action in clinical practice does not "just naturally" follow. Like novices in any practice, student nurses often focus on one thing at a time, relying on deliberative problem solving, explicit tasks, and immediate patient needs and thus missing the clinical situation as a whole. To recognize the salience or relevance of patients' signs and symptoms as possible indications for treatment or other action, students need a perceptual grasp and narrative understanding of the nature of specific clinical situations.

As the student uses knowledge in situations of practice, she gains new understanding of and access to that knowledge, such as knowing how, when, and why it is relevant in particular situations. The student learns the ability to *use* knowledge by increasing her understanding of what practical clinical situations mean and increasing her facility for situated cognition, as well as thinking in action. By this we mean the student increases her cognitive capacities to think in relation to the particular demands of a situation. What is essential for nursing educators is helping students make the connections between acquiring and using knowledge. We call this *teaching for a sense of salience*.

Having a sense of salience—being able to recognize what is more or less important in a clinical situation—is the beginning point for clinical reasoning within a situation. Novice first-year students learn to prioritize actions, reflect on what they have learned from their experience, and improve the care they give on their next care assignment. Eventually this process of experiential learning over time creates a sense of salience about familiar clinical situations, and the student no longer has to deliberate on all priorities; some are just *obvious* on the basis of similarities of their prior experiential learning. This kind of repeated clinical experience is required in order to develop a growing differentiated sense of priorities in nursing practice, what we call a sense of salience.

Teaching for a sense of salience must be undertaken in the context of particular situations and requires that the teacher present experiential learning opportunities, a strategy called *situated teaching*. Whether the teacher and students are with a patient or in a classroom, the nurse educator coaches the students toward what is salient (most notable and significant) about a specific clinical situation and guides them to mine their knowledge to determine what actions they will take, thus helping them to develop clinical imagination and the skills of clinical reasoning.

We noted that in clinical settings, teachers guide and coach students to use clinical reasoning, to make a type of translation from knowledge needed for nursing practice, whether physiological, relational, or pharmacological, to concerns about a particular patient. As one educator explained, "If we are asking a question about heart failure we're not going to ask: 'What's the difference between right-sided and left-sided heart failure physiologically?' We're going to ask a question about how a nurse would care for a patient in left-sided heart failure. We would ask,

'What would be the concerns?' and the student would be expected to know that care would be designed primarily around respiratory issues."

We repeatedly observed such an approach in clinical settings, and although nurse educators tend to lump many kinds of reasoning and action strategies under a loosely construed and extraordinarily broad notion of "critical thinking," their actual clinical teaching strategies are more differentiated and rooted in particular situations. Questioning and engaging students in dialogue are effective ways of integrating and developing students' knowledge, skilled know-how, and ethical comportment while guiding students to grasp the salience of a clinical situation. As the students develop a sense of salience and skill, teachers can modify these strategies so that the students can increasingly rely on their own clinical imagination and clinical reasoning.

In this paradigm case, we focus on Diane Pestolesi who guides her students to a sense of salience through examples from particular patients. A midcareer nurse educator, Pestolesi teaches at Saddleback Community College, a commuter school in Southern California, and practices at a local hospital.

5

PARADIGM CASE

DIANE PESTOLESI, PRACTITIONER AND TEACHER

I teach the fourth semester. By the time students get to fourth semester and they're assessing patients and dealing with families in crisis, it's essential that they've honed their communication skills and their ability to identify subtle changes in behavior in a client who's acutely ill because, as we talked about, for example, last week, the level of consciousness is the most sensitive indicator of the deterioration of neurological status. Well, if they don't know normal behavioral kinds of responses patients would have from a pathological condition, they would never pick up on these little changes. So it's foundational, I think, for them to be able to pick up on those changes and find subtle changes in patient assessment by knowing normal behavior.

DIANE PESTOLESI, who teaches in both the classroom and clinic, is energetic, reflective about her practice, and confident about her abilities. In the classroom, Pestolesi connects her practice as a critical care nurse to her clinical teaching. The focus of the class is on a clinical situation, and Pestolesi engages the students in solving clinical puzzles. As she teaches, she strides around the classroom, asking questions or fielding comments from her students. She speaks with confidence, in paragraphs, firing off questions in rapid bursts.

Yet she is skilled at knowing when to temper herself, as for example when she is speaking one-on-one with a student in clinical. In these situations, she tries "not to be authoritarian or threatening. Hard to do, I'm six feet tall; most of them are not," said Pestolesi, who sits down with her students and tries "to minimize the negative impact that I would have on their clinical performance."

Pestolesi readies herself for the classroom by reviewing the material and making decisions: "To make sure I was familiar with all my lecture notes, the PowerPoint, and my case study for burns, I reviewed it again, highlighted some key points that I wanted to bring out to show them how it related back to shock so that we could build on what they knew already. I spent a little extra time [questioning students] just to make sure that I had a clear idea of where we're starting and where we needed to get to by the end."

The notion of having a clear starting and ending point also guides Pestolesi in thinking about the entire course. For example, speaking about teaching students who have some experience with advanced medical-surgical topics, she explains, "Introduction to Professional Development is my way of taking what I think are the key concepts that a beginning nurse needs and making them applicable, making them something that they own, and making them come alive, too . . . not to overwhelm them with jargon but to ply them with bottom-line information that an associate's degree nurse needs to begin to practice safely and competently."

Pestolesi understands that she cannot possibly teach everything that her students will need to know to practice: "There's no one who could possibly present to them everything that they need to know about advanced med/surgical nursing in the time that we have allotted together." Characteristic of master teachers, she focuses on what she wants the students to learn, taking an approach that she describes by paraphrasing the football coach John Wooten: "It's what you learn after you know it all that really counts." With that neat statement, she encapsulates her teaching: a cumulative, iterative practice, in which she would like her students to learn to formulate questions, to be curious, to wonder whether they have enough information about clinical situations, and to reflect on their experiences.

Drawing from Practice

Whether in the classroom or in a clinical situation, Pestolesi draws directly on her experiences in practice, bringing them to the center. She does not simply mention her practice in her classes; she uses her practice experiences as organizing principles for the class: "What we see in clinical most of the time almost dictates the organization of what we present in class." As she explains, her practice in intensive care shapes what she emphasizes:

I currently practice in intensive care, Orange County, and one of the main things that's influenced the way that I teach is what I see in clinical practice. And so I have emphasized the things that I think we see most of the time with most of the patients and de-emphasize things that I would consider to be minutiae. I've also increased the use of technology because I see that in practice as well and because I think there's so much good information out there. I think the use of technology (what's available out there) and what I see in clinical practice have been probably the two big things that have influenced how I teach the course.

When Pestolesi interprets her practice world for her students, she goes beyond telling them what to expect on the clinical unit or warning them about potential pitfalls. As she teaches, she recognizes, names, organizes, and conveys what she sees and does in practice in ways that enable students to imagine what she is seeing and talking about. Integrating her clinical experiences with the material the students encounter in the classroom, "I try to help make connections," Pestolesi explains, "between what we're learning in 'theory' and what they might see in clinical."

Cases, Vignettes, and Stories

In the classroom, Pestolesi always returns to practice to guide students toward what they need to know. She reinforces experiential learning from clinical in the classroom and teaches for a sense of salience by using stories and cases.

How do you make the connections of the experiential learning in the classroom? I do it through storytelling, case presentation, the problem-based learning.... I've increased the use of case studies as a teaching aid. I have a case study for every topic ... oftentimes a few. But anytime I stop and tell a story ... I always get positive feedback ... because it's what makes it stick, it makes it come alive to them, it makes them see their patients that day in class. And when other students bring the subject up, too, it's another perspective and so when you can say, "This is how this applies," they [see that], "OK, there's more than one way to do this." My goal is to show them, yeah, this is the rule, this is what we're supposed to do, but this allows them to critically think, understanding the complex pathophysiology that goes into it.

One way Pestolesi makes connections between practice and pathophysiology or pharmacology is by saying, "'Technically, now this is what you're supposed to see.' And then I'll say, 'Just the other day I had a gentleman who. . .' and describe him. My goal in the stories and the descriptions is to paint a picture for them and to make it come alive and to make them understand the thought processes that I go through and the decisions that are made in treatment." By describing how she thinks about a patient, Pestolesi models for students how she sifts and sorts all the details of taking care of patients, the pieces of information, laboratory results, doctor's orders, and nursing notes.

She is also candid about her experience. One of the cases that Pestolesi gives her students is the story of a serious error she made just after finishing nursing school:

> I was to give Synthroid IV to a woman who was hypothyroid. The order . . . I thought was a very large dose. When the vials came up, there were three vials to be reconstituted, which again made me think that this is too large of a dose. So I called the pharmacy, and the pharmacist said, "Well, it is a large dose, but it is within the possible range of dosages." I had this icky feeling that it wasn't right.
>
> I went to the patient, and as I was pushing the IV med in, again, I had this icky feeling that it was the wrong dose. So, I then went back to the chart and looked at the original doctor's order, which I had not done, but should have done from the beginning.
>
> It was an error . . . I had given three times the amount of the drug that was intended.
>
> I went hot and cold. I thought, "Well, this is the end of my nursing career. I will lose my license." I called the doctor and told him about the error. "I am really sorry, I have made a terrible medication error. I gave your patient three times the dosage of Synthroid that was ordered. What can I do to help this patient?" He said to watch her closely for arrhythmias, to carry Inderal in my pocket, ready to administer it to her if she had a tachycardia.
>
> I arranged with the other nurses to watch my other patients while I stayed in the patient's room. The patient became very antsy, very hot then, and for the first time after surgery needed to have a bowel movement. The patient dramatized all the symptoms of hyperthyroid. I fanned the patient. I put a cool cloth on her head, and stayed with her. Her pulse stayed below 120.
>
> She came through it without arrythmias, but I will never give the wrong dose of Synthroid again. I will always check the original order and call the doctor if I have questions. I will never go against my

instincts, overriding my icky feeling that this is not right. I learned that I could survive and continue to be a nurse, even though I made a terrible error. I am grateful that the patient came through OK. I filled out an incident report at the end of the shift.

What is striking about the account was that she remembers how she felt, the dread of having her license revoked, the fear she felt for her patient, the recognition that while she was preparing the medication there was something that was not right, and her attention to the patient, in particular what the patient was experiencing.

She explained one of the reasons she uses her own story: "It makes it OK, in a sense, because they put you on this [pedestal]: 'Oh, you never made a med error.'" In telling her story, Pestolesi's goal is to teach students how to prevent errors as well as how to respond to errors when they occur. She emphasizes honesty and integrity, admitting the error immediately and staying with her patient. She also uses the example to illustrate hyperthyroidism, its presentation and the experiences of the patient: "I describe to them how a patient became hyperthyroid because of my medication error and how we handled it. They all get the hyperthyroid questions correct on the test."

The story illustrates that emotion has cognitive content and is intertwined with perception (Folkman & Lazarus, 1982; Merleau-Ponty, 1962). For example, the students can hear the foreboding sense in Pestolesi's voice when she contemplates the dangers to her patient. Her detailed focus on the patient's every symptom indicates what should be attended to in this situation. The relief in her voice in relaying the good outcome also reinforces the significance and risk of the thyroid overdose. As it became clear that the patient safely weathered the induced thyroid "storm" from the overdose, Pestolesi's sense of pride and relief over a responsibility well met demonstrates that "doing the right thing" is its own reward; she embodies the truth that acting responsibly in the face of a medication error is the best and only option.

Pestolesi's story is, ultimately, about embodying the practice of nursing. The students could read a moral compass in her responses, her tone of voice, and what she was concerned about. She cautions them not to override their intuition. Identifying with her, the students see a moral vision of ethical comportment. Remorse and regret are expressed, but not guilt, self-recrimination, or perfectionism. While teaching the students to be honest and courageous when the worst happens, she is also teaching them, firsthand, that they can survive the "mistake" if they act with integrity and with a primary concern for the patient.

Just as she weaves stories and cases from practice in and out of her classes and clinical sessions, in our interviews Pestolesi constantly shifted between examples about her classroom teaching and her clinical instruction. Her facility in shifting between the worlds marks her teaching and allows her students in the classroom to imagine being with a patient on a medical-surgical floor, deciding what needs to be done next and why. She helps her students develop their clinical imagination by inviting them to stand beside her, see the patient, read the laboratory results, try to understand what the patient is experiencing, and make judgments about what the patient needs.

In the classroom, Pestolesi uses case studies as a point of departure for discussion about pathophysiology, and she engages her students in sharing with each other their experiences with patients. Explaining the importance of bringing concerns for particular patients into the classroom, Pestolesi describes her approach:

> Next week, we're talking about endocrine; we have a couple of endocrine case studies. The purpose is not to go over the case studies verbatim, but to compare the case with what the student has experienced in clinical. The topic is endocrine so [we have to hope] our students had some patient with big endocrine problems. As you've gone on through your clinical day, as the faculty member you know what every person's been involved with in clinical. So I frequently will have the person who had the patient on insulin or in adrenal crisis talk about what the patient looked like and what was the priority and why they did this and how that happened. The whole goal is to tie that back to theory [the classroom material] and bring that patient to life for those students who didn't have the opportunity to take care of that patient. So [the students] go through their own experiences first; they'll share around the table. Then we'll go through a more structured approach to the case studies; they've had the case studies before class and they'll go through them and work them out and that helps them to bring the patient to life and maybe nobody that week had a good endocrine patient and so it's sort of our back-up plan, to reinforce the theory [the classroom material] in clinical practice.

By asking her students to relate their experiences, Pestolesi is asking them to articulate their sense of practice. This is another way for students to learn to reflect on their care. Articulating her own practice—what she does, how she practices, and why—is also what she must do in order to organize the topics of her classes, present information, and emphasize points in her teaching. Both of these interpretive pedagogical strategies help Pestolesi teach her students to develop a sense of salience in a clinical situation.

Pestolesi also uses patient examples or cases in part because she believes that students are more engaged during the class:

> I've taken some of those concepts and integrated them into the pathophysiology-based part because I find that the students are much more engaged when we're talking about patho and applying it to critically ill patients. So for example, the first test that we had covered cardiovascular, EKG, ACLS [advanced cardiac life support], cardiac dysfunction, including the pathophysiology, but it also covered leadership styles.
>
> It leads them through a case where it shows this very authoritarian style of leadership. And it just asks simple case study questions: What kind of leadership style was this? What kind of leader are you? We do exercises on the different kinds of leadership styles. I include delegation and feedback, talking about being an EMT in an ICU and having to delegate. If they don't know what the acute care, unlicensed assistant personnel can do, they must look it up on the hospital Website.

Pestolesi stated that she believes students are more engaged with the pathophysiology she is teaching when she illustrates it from her own practice with particular critically ill patients. She involves her students in searching for answers not to rhetorical questions but to ones that require students to engage in inquiry. Just as in actual clinical practice, the inquiry can move in several directions. She is not looking for a single correct answer.

Pestolesi's students value her ongoing experience in practice as important to their learning. A skilled clinician, a practitioner who is able to anticipate "everything," she questions them before they try to do a procedure new to them. As one student said, "The fact that she's a nurse ... she works on weekends ... sets an example for me, at least, that she's in a setting, she knows. . . . So you can look up to her and what she's telling you and what she's doing and it's current and she knows and she's on top of it and she's very smart. She anticipates everything that comes and you can just tell she's very well skilled."

Knowing Her Students

Through her questioning of students in class, postclinical conference, and on the clinical unit, Pestolesi gets to know them, how they reason, and where they may need help or coaching. "What I care about is how you think about what you do," she tells them. As she explained to us, "and so it's important to try to understand how they think, to try to focus them on improving their critical thinking skills and to stimulate them to ask the next question." She offered the following example of how she learns how her students think from her clinical instruction:

> So I try to help make connections between what we're learning in theory [the classroom] and what they might see in clinical, based on my own clinical experiences as well as by presenting them with pieces that represent what they may see in clinical. For example, yesterday, in my clinical with my students, we did our version of a code blue [patient cardio-pulmonary resuscitation]. And for something a little different this time, I went around and I saw my students in clinical and I got an idea of what their patients are like and what they're doing for them . . . and each time when I had a student leading the code, I made the piece that they coded tailored to their clinical situation that day, and said, "OK, you're coming back from break and now your patient who's on a ventilator with renal failure does this. . . ." Not only do they have to think about the algorithm . . . they have to think of how it applies to their patient. So I was more patient with them and maybe prompted them just a little bit to think about things. But I'll tell you what. You learn who critically thinks well and you learn who problem-solves and you learn who can think on their feet and who can't. And by doing something like that, you learn so much about your students.

Pestolesi tailors her questions for her students by learning about their patients, figuring out what might need to be done, and giving them a scenario. She uses as examples the patients the students know, the ones they have cared for during the day, and asks what-if questions that build on the student's existing knowledge base. She is constantly pushing the students to take their thinking to the next step, the next level, to consider other dimensions of the problem that they have not thought of. But she does this skillfully, on the basis of knowing the student's abilities, background, and character, and always with a view of the kind of nurse she wants the student to become.

Pestolesi tries to help her students make the most of their education, and she is particularly concerned with those who come to nursing as a second career. "And they get that as an adult learner, what they need out of that to make it a successful experience. We don't predetermine what is good or not good, what is success or not success. It's, 'What did you learn, what would you change, how would you do it over again?' We give them a lot of control over where they go with it."

By knowing how her students think, as a clinical instructor Pestolesi has a sense about when to press them to try a procedure or skill and when to stop pressing them. "Because I always feel like I'm going to push them a little step farther … but I don't want to push them off the cliff." She knows their limits and their strengths: "So we try to take it from the basic to the more complex and we try to allow them the ability to direct that as much as they can, with us overseeing it so that it's safe and appropriate." By insisting that students start with the simple and move on to more complex practices or ideas, she has a good idea about whether they understand the whole clinical picture of a patient, including the pathophysiology, pharmacology, nursing theory, and social or behavioral theories.

Coaching

Part of Pestolesi's success in teaching for a sense of salience comes from her finely tuned ability to coach her students. Most often used in the clinic setting, coaching involves encouraging students, giving them advice, and asking them a series of questions before they take care of a patient. A good coach helps students overcome their anxiety so that they can demonstrate their best practice. A good coach tailors the coaching to the particular student and the particular situation. Pestolesi is an effective coach in the clinical setting, because she knows her students and because she teaches from a deep background understanding of the practice. She has a reliable understanding of most open-ended clinical situations. She is also reflective about her approach and its impact on the student.

In all this, she tries to be what she calls a "nonfactor," by which she means asking students questions in a nonthreatening way:

> My goal in the clinical area is to be a nonfactor, just to be there … trying not to be authoritarian … trying to get them to offer up information. For example, [with a] weak student, I just ask, "Well, tell me what you see. What do you see?" I try to guide without telling. Try to leave them with a, "OK, then you … " I also have this little thing that I do frequently: "OK, then your question for the morning is, why, blah, blah, blah? And try not to ask the nurses, OK? This is *your* question." So that it's more like … "OK, see what you can find out about this. Check the chart and look for something about that that is going to help you understand this. It'll make everything click and you'll totally get it."

By being a nonfactor, Pestolesi is trying not to add additional stress for the student by her presence. She strives to be positive and encouraging, helping to bring out the student's knowledge and skill by asking questions that point the student toward understanding the nature of the particular clinical situation.

Pestolesi also offers direct guidance. In an exchange we observed between Pestolesi and a student who was preparing a drug dose, Pestolesi's ability to offer guidance in a nonthreatening way was evident. Pestolesi and the student talked through each step of reconstituting the drug and measuring the correct dosage. Both Pestolesi and her student asked questions and clarified each other's thinking.

Teaching from Her Stance in Practice

Guided by what she believes is ultimately good for the patient, Pestolesi coaches her students toward patient-centered learning. In her advanced medical-surgical nursing class, Pestolesi uses situated teaching, where she draws on narrative, the patient's context, and interpretation about the patient's situation. In particular, she questions her students to help them enrich their abstract understanding of textbook accounts with their newly gained understanding of clinical situations. They can then use this enriched knowledge to inform responses in future clinical situations. Her questions help students clarify the nature of the situation. In particular, she helps the less-experienced student grasp what is most salient in the unstructured clinical situation and facilitates the student's decision about what ought to take the highest priority.

Keeping patient safety paramount, she takes time to bring the student along. As Pestolesi put it, "I feel like I'm on a little mission and I try to make [the exchange] more about 'We need to know this . . . we're working together to get this information for them,' rather than 'I'm testing to know if you know the information.' I'm trying to encourage them to use critical thinking in the clinical area without calling it critical thinking, without punishing them if they don't get it. Rather, I'm making the journey, the process, something that they get comfortable with so they continue to ask questions."

Pestolesi's high expectations for her students earn their respect for her. One student told us that she tapes Pestolesi's lectures and listens to them when she takes walks. Pestolesi holds students accountable for their education: "One of my assumptions that I make, and I share with the students, is that you need to take responsibility for your own learning. I can lead you to water but I can't make you drink." She emphasizes that the students are responsible for their learning, in school and after they graduate. She also asks them "to direct" their own learning: "So I make sure that they understand that it is their responsibility to take ownership of the process and do their reading and do whatever preparation they take that might be different from the other guy, in order to acquire the knowledge that is necessary to pass the course."

Similarly, Pestolesi also demands that students be engaged with her and each other in the classroom:

> I make them a little more accountable and try to go away from spoon feeding ... if you've looked through the syllabus, you see we've got complete lecture notes and we put it all on Blackboard and they just pull it up at home and print it. The intent of that is so that they don't sit there when we're in class and just scratch down notes one after another; so that they really can engage and that they can really participate in the discussion and then are held responsible for already having reviewed those notes and readings and that kind of thing; so that they're prepared to participate fully in class.

Pestolesi expects her students to be proactive, seeking out ways to learn: "They need to actively seek out and get involved with those things that surround them. I always tell them, because I take a great deal of personal pride in the fact that my students are proactive and are involved and don't shy away, 'Don't sit back and hope that you can learn one day, maybe. Put yourself out there. Take a risk, get involved, be safe, but don't hesitate to seek out experiences whenever you're in the clinical area.'"

Pestolesi is able to maintain her high expectations of students in part because her colleagues share those same expectations. A colleague told a story about a student who could not figure out why a patient had been in the hospital for seven days after an appendectomy. After some investigation, the student learned that the patient had gangrene in the colon. The instructor described what then happened in postclinical conference: "We had a great big, long conversation in postclinical conference that day about the power of an inquisitive mind ... if something isn't textbook, then we really should be doing some more delving into why the patient's there and what is this medication for if it has nothing to do with what we think the patient is there for, to have a little bit more inquisitiveness about searching out why something is going on or what's happening with the patient. And again, it's experience. The more they learn, the more those things will pop up as red flags."

Continuing to ask questions is, to Pestolesi and her colleagues, a core professional responsibility. Thus Pestolesi sees the goal of her teaching not as simply covering a lot of material in each class but as guiding her students. By asking her students to draw on their knowledge of pathophysiology, pharmacology, or social and behavioral science, she models the type of integrative learning that she would like her students to be engaged in for the rest of their careers: "This responsibility and accountability for lifelong learning is very important to us. If you're out there in the clinical area and you don't know how to do something and we see you not seeking out resources to fill that knowledge gap, that's really serious to us. That is not meeting objectives. On that alone [not looking up needed information], it is possible that a student could not progress to preceptorship."

Pestolesi explained the importance of being confident that students can practice safely without supervision:

> Our goal is not to let students who would be still, perhaps, dangerous to patient safety . . . to preceptorship . . . so we're very careful. This is our last, last thing before they get to be nurses so . . . we're very serious about who we let get through. . . . As they're moving through this progression from student to nurse, the rope we give them gets a little bit longer and we wean them from us, as best we can, while they're gaining enough confidence to keep on walking . . . and then ultimately using us and the nurse they're preceptoring with less and less. Our civic responsibility and our own professional accountability to our practice and the patients in the world is really important to us. And so the moderately dangerous students usually we've picked up on, and we're essentially ensuring that they won't progress to the less supervised preceptorship experience, because we communicate clearly with them.

One striking aspect of this comment is the absence of any mention of the national licensing examination. The separation between "student" and "nurse" is not a passing score on the NCLEX-RN, but the judgment that the person is prepared to practice. Another is emphasis on civic responsibility. Pestolesi and her colleagues are deeply concerned about those they allow to enter the profession. One reason is their strong sense of integrity, their sense of responsibility for the profession; another is their sense of duty to the school. Pestolesi, the consummate practitioner, fears the specter of a "moderately dangerous" student who may harm patients and who runs counter to her professional identity as a practitioner and educator.

In the following chapter, we look in greater detail at four of Pestolesi's key strategies for teaching in both classroom and clinical setting: building on prior knowledge, using questions, giving her students opportunities to rehearse their knowledge for use in practice, and reflecting on their practice. The result is that she supports her students in developing a sense of salience and a rich clinical imagination.

6

STRATEGIES FOR TEACHING FOR A SENSE OF SALIENCE

WHETHER TEACHING in the classroom or clinical setting, Pestolesi uses a range of strategies, tailoring her teaching to the situation as well as to her students and their particular clinical experience. We noted, moreover, that she demonstrates how nursing educators can focus on developing students' sense of salience and situated use of knowledge. In observing Pestolesi's teaching and that of other nurse educators, we found that four strategies are particularly effective in helping students appropriately use knowledge and over time develop a sense of salience. First, she teaches by building on what students have already learned in other classes and introduces new knowledge that she expects students to integrate. For example, she will introduce pathophysiology of heart disease for adults and then discuss the pathophysiology of heart failure in older patients. She cycles back to introducing and building on what students have already learned. Second, she guides student thinking by posing questions relevant to particular patient situations. Third, she helps students rehearse for practice by giving them an opportunity to express their ideas for, approaches to, and possible complications in caring for a patient. Fourth, through questions and high expectations for their understanding of patient situations, she guides them in their reflection on practice.

Creating Continuity and Coherence in Learning

"The whole course is sort of designed around that concept as well, simple to complex, single topics to integration of topics," explains Pestolesi, "single pathology to the integration of complex pathology to complex pathology that doesn't follow the rules so that it is even atypical in its complexity."

In moving "from simple to complex," she starts,

> at a very kind of a basic level … what you need to know most to what you might not see as frequently.… For example, the first couple of weeks I spend talking about EKGs [electrocardiograms] and ACLS [advanced cardiac life support] type algorithms and treatment for those types of things because every single patient in this area, with few exceptions, requires EKG monitoring and has potential for requiring some advanced cardiac life supportive medications, treatments, or interventions. So that's what we start with and we go right from there to respiratory failure and things of that nature.

Along the way, she teaches students the language of nursing and widens the scope of classroom discussions from situations that occur with frequency to those that are less frequent. She starts with a discussion of what she sees as common illnesses or problems, introducing first what will become familiar early in the students' practices and moves on to less common occurrences of problems or illnesses. Then, as students gain experience, Pestolesi continues, always building on what students have already experienced and anticipating what they will experience.

Pestolesi iteratively reviews and builds on materials, drawing on what students have already learned or experienced in her class and other courses. For example, in describing a class on shock, Pestolesi explains how she builds students' knowledge and understanding by tying topics together:

> We went through shock and talked about tissue perfusion perspective … and related it back to when we had talked about EKG, dysrhythmias, cardiac dysfunction and low cardiac output syndrome, what cardiogenic shock looked like, from a low cardiac output perspective [pump failure] and compared shock now and a tissue perfusion problem, comparing the similarities between what they already knew from a couple of weeks ago when they studied how shock from blood loss is a similar type of problem with tissue perfusion, the concept that we are covering now with heart failure. And then I went on to say, "So if we know that shock is a tissue perfusion thing, let's back up and figure out what caused it."

Pestolesi creates coherence through explicit ties between old and new, reinforcing what students already know and clearly identifying significant distinctions in the new situation: "We talked about cardiogenic shock. [I said] 'You already know that it's a pump problem. Now let's talk about other causes. We can have a pump problem, we can have a volume problem, we can have a distribution problem.' And then we went from that perspective."

Explaining why she deliberately weaves the old with the new, pointing out what she has already introduced, briefly reviewing it, and then moving on to new material, Pestolesi says that her goal is helping students structure their understanding of the salience of the clinical situation. Speaking of a particular portion of the class, she said, "Knowing we had to cover a lot, I was afraid that if I didn't make strong ties to what they already knew, they would feel overwhelmed with the volume of information. I tried to make strong ties with what they knew. It seemed to flow really pretty well, and they were very engaged, answering questions: 'Oh, we would need vasoconstrictors,' 'We would need after load reducers,' 'We would need volume expanders.'"

Is the problem a pump or heart failure problem, a volume distribution problem, or a problem of low volume? What the nurse does depends on what the problem is, so she must sort out the salient aspects of the situation accurately in order to grasp the nature of the problem. For example, it would be disastrous to add volume to a patient who is in shock due to heart failure but essential for a patient in shock due to low blood-fluid volume. Pestolesi coaches students on recognizing and understanding the salient differences in these situations.

Missed Opportunities for Learning

Like Pestolesi, other educators weave old and new as they guide students in clinical settings. We noted this strategy, along with staging, is often used in the first year, when students work on mastering one new clinical skill at a time, as three first-year nursing students explained:

STUDENT 1: We just had focused clinical on medication administration.

STUDENT 2: Different weeks we'll study different things in lecture and then we'll have a focus . . . last week was documentation, this week is medication administration. Whatever we learn in lecture then we bring it into clinical, and it usually covers about a week. Medication administration is two weeks, so that's about four clinical days.

STUDENT 1: And they build on each other so you do each thing.

STUDENT 2: You retain. You do the same thing you did last week plus this and then plus that. So you can't just drop [what] you've learned; you have to keep it going the whole time.

STUDENT 1: You're assigned a patient and this time we'll be giving medication.

STUDENT 2: Whereas before we didn't do that. . . ..

STUDENT 1: We just did the assessment and documentation . . . something is added.

STUDENT 3: It's like a scheduled introduction: one scary experience is added per clinical experience.

The third student's comment, "one scary experience is added per clinical experience," highlights the importance of building knowledge to make the high-stakes clinical environment more manageable during the first year of clinical learning.

Although the ability to break down complex tasks into their components, simplify them, and teach element by element is useful and even necessary for teaching novices, we found that nurse educators often take simplification too far. In skills lab, students learn many isolated clinical procedures, communication skills, and the performance of various tasks by having all the elements identified and then practicing one element at a time. For example, we observed the task of assembling an IV pump with a medication to be titrated broken down into a step-by-step process, as were many procedures such as inserting a Foley catheter, or teaching patients about caring for themselves at home after discharge. The simplification of tasks is not adequate preparation for grasping the nature of whole complex clinical situations, where students must take into account a patient's current situation, such as the interrelationships of therapies or multiple diseases. Finally, the situation is too complex to think of it in terms of elements or parts alone.

Pestolesi moves beyond simplification and takes an integrative approach that demands that her students respond to real clinical situations by drawing on what they learned in their reading and in the classroom. In her classroom and clinical teaching, Pestolesi helps her students integrate the knowledge they are learning in order to use it appropriately in the clinical setting. Aware that the students have not learned theoretical knowledge or science until they put it into use in practice, she does not—indeed, cannot—separate knowledge and practice into discrete compartments. Her teaching reflects her understanding that knowledge and practice are dialogical, tightly woven with each shaping the other. Whether in the classroom or clinical setting, she offers opportunities for students to learn from their own or the instructor's clinical experience and from situations as they evolved in the clinical setting. Thus she addresses the whole of the clinical situation and helps students learn what must guide them in their decisions for action.

Using Questions

Just as in the clinical setting, situated questioning is an effective teaching strategy in the classroom. The process serves as a diagnostic tool, a way to see how students are thinking, and a way to guide students toward a sense of salience and the ability to engage their clinical reasoning. Pestolesi always asks the students a series of questions that they need to answer before they can proceed. As Pestolesi explains, through a series of specific, unambiguous questions to find out what her students believe about their patients, she also makes evident to them the many pieces of information they must take into account in making decisions for action. "I have found that there are students who don't see it when it's right in front of them and have to be guided step-by-step to dissect it down to its very component parts," she explains, "and other students, who, if you say, 'Tell me,' have seen it all already and written it up."

Pestolesi describes how she asks students to articulate what they know about a patient, in this case about the patient's respiratory status, and how, depending on the student's answer, she will prompt the student to "dissect down" and thus make the assessment:

> I say, "Tell me about your patient. What are you doing today?" They say, "Well, he's this, he's that"...and start to describe what the patient is like. And perhaps I'll ask a question: "Well, how's his respiratory status?" If they say, "Well, it's fine," I might say, "Now, let's back up for a second and tell me, what do you see that makes you tell me that it's fine?" so that they can dissect down to the nth degree with little bits of information that they have assembled in their head that tell them that the patient's respiratory status is fine...no increased breathing, the respiratory rates are within normal, their color is pink, their oxygen saturation is good, the lung sounds like this...I force them to revisit all those things that they did, assimilated or not.

As Pestolesi takes the students step-by-step through their thinking about their patients, a missed or wrong answer prompts her to ask questions that unearth where the student made a wrong assumption or did not know information. Pestolesi is aware of the potential embarrassment that her questions may provoke in a student, but she does not shy away from questioning. She sees her questioning as essential to the students' learning. As another teacher who uses questions in a similar way noted, if the students do not know the answer to a question, she asks them "knowledge-based questions on material that's been covered in the current or previous course," leading them to the answer. "They're almost always surprised when they realize they do know the answer; they just need to be shown how to find it." This is an example of teaching students to recognize and use relevant knowledge in a particular situation.

Pestolesi's students appreciate her style of questioning: "Professor Pestolesi is very strong on that. She says no one is inferior if they're learning. And everybody learns. And as long as you can learn, you're going to be a success. It's when you don't want to learn that there's a problem."

Guiding Students Toward a Sense of Salience

Once students learn to grasp the major concerns in a situation, they can put some order and priorities to the list of tasks that need to be accomplished, such as, "I am primarily concerned about the patient's respiratory status this morning, so I am going to focus on having the patient deep-breathe and cough, as well as position her for good air exchange."

Pestolesi's account of an exchange with a student in the ICU demonstrates how instructors can use guiding questions to help students learn to discern the most important concerns and prioritize action:

> I had a student in a critical care environment with a patient who was a little lady, eightyish. She was admitted to the ICU for urosepsis. The student did a write up on this patient, about a five-page preclinical workup. Early on in the shift, maybe 8:30, I asked, "Tell me what your patient's priority of care will be today." She said, "altered urinary elimination." Well, the lady had gone from her admission diagnosis ten days before with urosepsis into acute respiratory distress syndrome, had to be intubated, mechanically ventilated, and was finally weaned off the ventilator the day before . . . they were so concerned that the lady would not be able to stay off the ventilator that the vent was still in the room. The lady had been trached the day before as well. She had the humidified air set up to her trach tube going.

So I said, "Now tell me why you chose that." "Well, she came in with urosepsis." I said, "OK. Now, when you look at this lady, what do you see?" "She's a frail little lady." "OK. Tell me what you see that makes you concerned for this lady enough to keep her in the ICU. What's keeping her here?" "Well, hmm..." And she had to think. I said, "Remember when we talked about her PAO2 this morning?" She said, "Yeah." I said, "What was it?" She said, "52." I said, "OK. So does that concern you?"

I had to really back up and go step-by-step. Finally, I said, "And she had already had rounds with the intensivist, who asked, 'How are her secretions? How often are we suctioning her? Do you think they could handle her on the floor?'"

The student didn't pick up on any of those clues. So I said, "What was your PAO2 again and what's keeping her in the ICU?" I'm trying not to make her totally embarrassed or ashamed about it, and she finally said, "Oh, yeah, it's the oxygenation issue." And I thought, "Holy smokes! I just had to take her back step-by-step, take her back, take her back." By now, we were standing in the patient's doorway, looking at her. "Now tell me what you see." So, needless to say, she had to work her way back through it and redo it and she came around and realized that it was her gas exchange issues that really were keeping her patient in the ICU.

With this example, Pestolesi describes how difficult it is for students to assess and understand the nature of the clinical situation for the patient. Because the student was accustomed to reading about the patient's condition in the chart, she was more focused on the clear write-up in the chart about the patient's urosepsis ten days ago than her current acute respiratory problems. Although such practical misinterpretation of a clinical situation is shocking to Pestolesi as an expert nurse, she is patient with the student and uses the student's inability to grasp the situation as a starting point in helping the student to see the most salient aspects of the current situation.

Modeling a Lifelong Pursuit of Knowledge

In questioning her students to find out what they know or how they think about a problem, Pestolesi also models a way of thinking about practice: start from what one knows or can see and then move on to what information needs to be found, tested for, or uncovered. For example, Pestolesi furnished a follow-up on the student whose patient had the oxygenation problem:

> Last week she came to clinical and, of course, she was one of the first people I saw because I'm concerned about the student not seeing what to me seems so obvious...with much trepidation said, "Tell me about your patient." And she was so right on. I even started looking at her paperwork and said, "This is great. Wow!" And I said, "Please don't be offended. Did you write this yourself? Did you really write this?" And she said, "Yeah, I did." I said, "This is 180 degrees from what you did last week. How did you do this? Why is this?" And she said, "Because I didn't get what you were really asking me. I didn't get what I was really supposed to do." But I didn't quite understand her.
>
> The student then elaborated: "When I was putting down what the priority patient problem was, I thought 'I have to know for sure,' so I had to see urosepsis. It was on the chart. Somebody else told me that that was a problem. I didn't realize that I could just look at her current patient problem and figure it out. When I went in to do my preclinical, I just looked and I said just what you asked me: 'What's keeping this patient in the critical care unit? Why is she still here?'"
>
> I thought, as an instructor, that's so simple, but it made that big of a difference to this student. So, those are the kinds of things that I lock in my head: "OK, remember this, for every student, every time."

When Pestolesi asked the student to reflect on her learning, the student explained that she had realized that the chart was only one piece of information that she needed to consult. She also needed to look at the patient and take in her behavior, skin color, the equipment that was in the room with the patient, and a whole host of other signs.

The student learned more from the experience than she might have if Pestolesi had supplied the answer, humiliated her, or reminded her to look beyond the chart. Her report of the second conversation with this student underscores the fruitfulness of her approach. It also points out her constant attempts to refine her teaching to "get it right." Realizing that many other students may use the same reasoning, in the future she will "remember this, for every student, every time." This is an a-ha moment for Pestolesi in her ongoing reflection on and growth in teaching.

Rehearsing for Practice

At the heart of clinical reasoning is the nurses' deep background knowledge: understanding of the nature of the particular situation bound as it is by time and context. Because this understanding is based on experiential learning (Bourdieu, 1990; Dreyfus, 1992; Dreyfus & Dreyfus, 1986), in a clinical situation the educators will often ask questions in advance to help the student ferret out what must be attended to on a particular day. Especially if the situation is too novel for the student, the teacher will have to frame the situation explicitly. It is highly risky to allow the student to discover too late, for example, that he or she should be attending to lung sounds, looking for early pulmonary edema (fluid in the lungs).

Preclinical Assignments: Preparing for Practice

Clinical teachers expect students to prepare for their patients, gathering a thorough understanding of the patient's history, course of illness and treatment in the hospital, all medications, and knowledge about possible contraindications, incompatibilities, and side effects.

This is a widespread practice. Almost all of the students in the Carnegie-NSNA survey reported having preclinical planning assignments. In their preclinical preparation, students often focus on medications: what possible drug interactions or side effects could occur, what to look for in terms of the patient's responses to the medications, and what laboratory results must be checked prior to giving medications. The students also outline the relevant pathophysiology and signs and symptoms that they might observe. Teachers question students about medications and the patient's clinical condition as the students prepare to administer the medication, or on their way to the patient's room.

When students arrive in the clinical setting with a prepared mind, they are in the best position to learn from underdetermined, open-ended clinical situations. They are ready to focus on salience and thus plan their care and anticipate their patient's concerns and needs, both of which are essential to clinical imagination. As one nurse educator explained, students are asked to discuss their expectations for the clinical assignment on the basis of their reading of the chart and references: "Lately we've started our morning with a conference and each student has been asked to identify what they think their priority of care is going to be for that day based on what they've done in their preparation and looking up everything about that client. And then we come to the postclinical conference and we say, 'OK, what was your priority and did it turn out that way?'"

In doing such extensive planning prior to each patient care assignment, students learn informally the limits of this planning because the high acuity of patients and short stays cause patients to change overnight or be discharged. Nevertheless, all the student groups and clinical educators we studied highly valued the experiential learning that came with students caring for one or two patients at a time.

What-If Rehearsing and Knowledge for Practice

Pestolesi creates opportunities for student to rehearse, drawing on their knowledge to make decisions in the face of ambiguous, open-ended clinical situations. She coaches her students to see and understand the nature of the context of the patient's current clinical condition, the immediate history, the most urgent current concerns, and why they are urgent or salient.

Pestolesi describes how she reinforces and deepens students' learning and sense of salience through such opportunities to rehearse decisions:

> Jennifer is a good theory [classroom] student and based on how she prepared for clinical I had a pretty good idea that she was very strong. She always had the right answers without my having to prompt her. . . . She'd draw correlations between complex pathophysiologic processes that are affecting the patient's presentation.
>
> She was at the head of the bed, describing what interventions would be appropriate for her patients . . . I thought, "I'll give her a harder scenario." Her patient in the CCU that day was somebody who was mechanically ventilated, had a pacemaker, who was put on C-Pap because they're trying to wean him from the ventilator. The patient had an insulin drip, and was having pacemaker problems and ventricular tachycardia problems as well.
>
> I said to her, "So, Jennifer, you get back from break, your patient, who has been pretty much unstable all day, kind of motions towards his chest . . . indicating some kind of discomfort or pain. You look up at the monitor and right in front of you, you see that he has gone into this." I put the rhythm on the screen, that little simulator. "That would sustain ventricular tachycardia. What are you going to do"
>
> Jennifer said, "Well, I would solicit help, activate ACLS. So I press the code blue button over the head of his bed and I'd be thinking, [primary] A, B, C, D survey. Airway, he's got his airways protected, he's on a vent. However, he's on C-Pap. . . . Well, C-Pap doesn't give him a rate, so I give him a rate but better yet, I take him off the ventilator, attach him to an ambu bag and begin to manually ventilate him to maximize his oxygenation."
>
> I'm thinking to myself, "She's really got it going." Then she proceeded to lead him right through the pulses V Pack, ventricular

fibrillation, ACLS algorhythm, without missing a beat. Also including in the fact that this gentleman had a pacemaker and that that
could have misfired and caused the V Tach to be set off...and this
was spontaneous, too. When she said to me at the end of the day, "I
was wondering if I could take my summer preceptor experience in the
ICU," you can imagine what my answer was: "They would be happy
to have you there."

Pestolesi's obvious delight in describing this student's readiness to
answer her questions speaks to the goals of her teaching. That this student
was able to answer every question appropriately indicated to Pestolesi that
the student was paying attention to the things a *nurse* would pay attention
to, and that the student had a clear grasp of the most salient aspects of the
patient's situation. In this particular case, posing what-if demonstrated to
Pestolesi and her student Jennifer that she is prepared.

Using Context

Pestolesi's pedagogical approach addresses the challenges common to
learning for complex, high-risk practices such as piloting an airplane or
practicing nursing, medicine, engineering, or law: how novice students
with no experience are ushered into the practice by "bootstrapping," as
the teacher carefully explains the risks, opportunities, and characteristics
of the practical situation in which he or she is placing the student. In
nursing, the student is prepared to enter clinical situations by extensive
preclinical preparation: looking up medications, studying pathophysiology, and reading the patient's medical and nursing history. However, in
the actual clinical situation the nurse educator may need to coach the student by remarking about the particulars of a patient's situation: "Today
we are no longer concerned about the patient's pneumonia because that
has resolved. But we are concerned about congestive heart failure due to
the resulting fluid in the patient's lungs. In addition, the patient is quite
anxious, awaiting his daughter to fly to the hospital."

We observed other clinical and classroom teachers, who like Pestolesi
help students contextualize and interpret clinical situations while coaching
them to make judgments or plans on their own. Rehearsing, as Pestolesi's
example suggests, helps students move toward that goal. In their precep-
torships, which occur in the fourth semester of their program, students
are given a 75 percent workload. By this time, Pestolesi begins to lead
them in less direct ways, asking other kinds of questions, such as, "Tell
me what you liked or didn't like and if you'd do it over again, what would

you do differently?" As she explains, "And our whole goal is for them to just kind of critically think about the day." She may make suggestions when she hears the students' accounts, "But most of the time, when they do that, it puts them in a place to ask the next question, critically think, figure out a strategy. So you really don't have to develop the strategy for them because they know what they're bringing to the picture and where they went wrong or why it didn't work out so well."

Whether they are being asked to rehearse how they will determine the salient features of a case or whether they are with the patient, students are increasingly focused on contextualizing the patient's current condition and disease trajectory. In clinical, their teachers do not break down situations or processes into simple elements; they use context to help students grasp the whole situation. Nurse educators often ask advanced students to compare a new clinical situation with a prior one, similar or contrasting. Pestolesi focuses on identifying the most salient aspects of the situation and then coaches the student to act and reason across changes in the particular situation over time.

Asking students to interpret specific clinical situations helps them understand types of illness and recognizable similarities among clinical situations. It helps students describe contrasts and similarities that point to *family resemblances* between patient clinical conditions rather than explicit signs and symptoms or elemental characteristics. The goals of these strategies are more holistic, in that they seek to help the student recognize the salience of the whole clinical situation.

Reflecting on Learning

Pestolesi's account of her student's struggle to grasp the salience of the elderly patient's situation and the student's subsequent examination of what she learned and how she took that knowledge back into practice serves as a model for the kind of reflection that we saw nursing educators routinely encourage in their students. Among the coaching strategies, one of the most prevalent was helping students reflect on their practice. The reflective strategies are shared within the community of learning and are typically "jointly owned," with one student's experience informing another. We found examples of postclinical reflection, whether in groups or with individual students, in all nine schools of nursing that we visited, and we found them to be extremely important. As they observe and reflect, pulling together what they learn in the clinical setting and other classes in taking care of patients, the students build and integrate knowledge, skilled know-how, and ethical comportment. The reflective pedagogies that nursing educators use to facilitate and articulate experiential learning are indeed a strength of nursing education and could contribute to other professions' educational processes.

Postclinical Conferences: Sharing Lessons Learned

After students finish their clinical assignments, they typically go to a clinical debriefing seminar to discuss their experiential learning for the day and how they plan to improve their care the next day. The clinical debriefings allow educators and students to mine the experiences of one student for the benefit of the whole group. We observed enthusiastic learning communities in daily postclinical conferences, with classmates assisting each other by carefully explaining what they had learned that week in clinical practice. Typically, students describe learning to do new procedures and working with patients with various diagnoses.

They also share with their classmates mistakes they have made. We noted that teachers asked students in advance of the conference whether or not they would feel comfortable talking about a near miss or mistake. If a student's patient is put at risk in any way (for example, through failure to check lab results prior to giving medications, an incorrect medication or dosage, injury, or inadequate isolation techniques), the student often reports this during the postclinical conference so that her colleagues can learn from her mistakes. Many students talk about how much easier the second day with the same patient is, and how they have managed to be more organized and effective because they have a better understanding of who the patient is and what his or her care needs are.

As observations suggest, there is solidarity in the learning communities around sharing lessons learned with classmates during clinical debriefing sessions:

NURSE EDUCATOR 1: They share with each other about their patients and what they did for the patients. They talk about what the particular challenges of the day were for them. I'm always impressed by how willing they are to share what didn't go well.

NURSE EDUCATOR 2: [laughing] That's right. They are. They are.

NURSE EDUCATOR 1: And they're really doing it to help the other students, you know? In other words, "Don't do what I just did today...." I look at it as a true learning experience. I don't expect them to hit the floor running. I want them to be prepared for clinical, but I don't expect clinical to be perfect. "So, it's not going to be a perfect day, but we're coming back tomorrow, you're going to have the same patient, tell me how you're going to do it differently."

Students are commonly asked about their plans for improvement for the second day of their clinical assignment. This expectation that students will reflect on their practice one day and try to improve on it a second day is the basis for a self-improving practice and was common to all the programs we visited. A nurse educator noted, "I have found that just having the students reflect about what they did puts them in a great place for the next day when they go back. They develop a goal to have something that motivates them and a specific objective that they've come to [by] themselves, through their critical reflection. That helps them to really own the process."

Many nurse educators agreed that having a bad day and reflecting on it and then successfully managing to do better the next day was far more useful to the student's development than to have an uneventful day with no challenges. We noted that one pervasive practice of situated, formative clinical assessment was reflecting with the students on day-to-day improvements of nursing practice.

A teacher described how she coaches students toward identifying areas of their practice that need improvement:

> When they walk out of a room and they've done something, you [say] ... "That was really good. Tell me what you would have done differently." Because rather than saying, "You didn't check her arm band, you didn't do this, you didn't do that," I always ask them to talk to me first because I want them to make the decision to critically think through what they just did and evaluate whether they would have changed anything. But our students get feedback on, I would say, almost a daily basis. Not written feedback but oral feedback on the unit. They get written feedback on their paperwork every single week. I have ten students; I probably spend, I would say, minimally, twenty, twenty-five hours a week grading their care plans that they turn in to me. I have changed from red to like aqua green or something like that because it looked like you bled all over their papers. But we really give feedback. "What did you think about this?" "In addition to what you wrote, could you think of anything else that might impact this patient?"

This teacher's dedication to feedback on students' reflection promotes a rich clinical learning environment, highly valuable to students because it focuses on concrete ways they can improve their practice. The teacher is aware that this feedback is more easily heard by students if it is done in less-threatening colors and framed in terms of questions that lead the student to a new line of thought, or if it assists them in integrating their classroom and clinical knowledge.

Because students learn in practice, they can—indeed, do—make inadvertent errors. In addition to learning the background knowledge needed to enter the practice area, learning the actual practice of nursing necessarily involves missteps. We noted on several occasions that if, during clinical, a student was on the way to making a mistake, the nurse educator would refrain from intervening until the last minute so that the student could experience as much independence as is responsibly possible and think through the procedure for herself. These moments are often the focus of postclinical discussions.

During clinical, teachers and students evaluate the performance of staff nurses and other health care colleagues, admiring some practice and rejecting other styles of practice. This too is discussed openly in postclinical conference debriefing sessions. Indeed, students value learning from reflection and readily volunteered their hard-won experiential knowledge, as this nurse educator recounted:

> The patient had difficulty breathing and the student wanted to give the meds instead of addressing the difficulty of breathing. Well, while we were sharing information about their patients, what they did that day, I didn't tell the student to say this, but she said, "I just want to tell you what I did today in clinical so you don't do the same thing, and here's what happened." Everybody's listening very attentively and they were asking her some questions. But she shared that. She didn't have to. I didn't tell her, "You must share that in postclinical conference," or anything like that, but she just went ahead and shared that, I guess, to reinforce what she had learned that day but also to benefit her fellow students in case that thing comes up with them.

The teacher's response to this student's honesty and generosity exemplifies her own approach in developing an open community of learning. Aware that focusing *only* on performance and on "being correct" prevents students from learning, she tries not to dampen students' curiosity and courage to learn experientially. This practice of sharing mistakes and near misses in clinical learning steeps students in an attitude of honesty about mistakes and creates a social contract that mandates disclosure, protecting patients as well as improving institutional systems of care. The common goal is to help others avoid making the same mistakes.

Experiential learning is facilitated by an open climate of learning in which students can discuss and examine transitions in understanding, including their false starts or misconceptions in actual clinical situations. This is a lifelong habit of the mind-set needed by all professionals if they are to become experts. The clinical conference is even more important as clinical placements for students become scarcer and students' exposure to many kinds of patients and diagnoses grows more difficult. As one student noted, by sharing their experiences students are able to relate varieties of patients and diagnoses that they would not otherwise get a chance to experience: "Our instructors encourage us to make connections between the classroom materials and the clinical experiences. They help increase our knowledge and facilitate our learning by helping us think through any tough situations with our patients and their diagnosis. They also encourage our peers to become involved, which increases the brainstorming and enriches the experience that each student gets to have."

Just as we found that teachers use the postclinical conference to help students learn and develop habits and values of professional practice, we observed that many nurse educators use assessments and pass-fail grading to encourage collaboration rather than competition for grades:

> We try not to single them out to embarrass them. We use it as a learning opportunity for the clinical group. I always ask the students if they can share their experience with the other members of the group.. . .Even if I don't think it's sensitive, they may be sensitive about it. If somebody brings up something in a weekly discussion forum, maybe it's not in clinical, and they were wrong on something. . .[we] try and correct them in a sensitive way since it could embarrass them. Then you can approach them on a one-on-one basis.

This approach to assessment helped to develop a sense of shared responsibility for learning from experience in communities of learning. Although we sometimes saw the postclinical conference debriefing time turned over for orientation to the unit, early in the quarter, and occasionally for didactic teaching of material that was not covered in class, this was an exception rather than a rule. We also found that some clinical nurses, hired as clinical instructors, seemed to lack understanding of the importance of "mining" and articulating experiential learning for the day, but again this was the exception. For the most part, nursing educators had a strong vision of using postclinical conferences to clarify and extend experiential learning and make the learning of one available to the whole clinical group. Thus, the postclinical conference was also an important site for integrating cognitive learning, skills of practice, and professional formation.

Using Narratives to Reflect on Practice

We observed that nurse educators highly value extension of knowledge from reflection on experience. Teachers used a variety of activities to help students discover, articulate, and share experiential clinical learning, whether during postclinical conferences or through comparisons between their preclinical planning and actual clinical experience.

Many instructors require students to write a narrative clinical journal chronicling their discoveries, growth, and lessons learned during clinical experiences. This nurse educator explains that the assignment helps focus the student on continuous improvement:

> [I ask] "So, based on what you wanted to accomplish today, how did it go?" "The next time you talked to a doctor were you able to . . . ?" and just to see if they really were able to implement the goals or the objectives that they set for themselves, helping them perhaps to strategize through, based on our clinical experience . . . "You might try this, you might try that." But most of the time, when they do that, it puts them in a place to ask the next question, critically think, figure out a strategy. So you really *don't* have to develop the strategy for them because they know what they're bringing to the picture and where they went wrong or why it didn't work out so well.

Narrative, first-person journals are usually not graded except for pass-fail, and most teachers give extensive written feedback, prodding students to think about ethical issues and question any possible knowledge gaps. In giving feedback to the students' narratives, teachers take care to avoid criticism or blame, and students take the observations and notes from the teachers seriously because they are a form of recognition and acknowledgment of the student's actual practice and particular struggles within the student's practice. This type of rich feedback is a powerful recognition of their practice that is far more telling than a letter grade.

Another nurse educator said that she consistently uses journals to tap into the student's experiential learning in ways that are similar to the group debriefing sessions: "Not taking away anything from your ability to start an IV or put in a catheter or anything else, but the brain is so much more important than the fingertips, [so] I give my students a communication sheet to fill out. . . . 'What was the best part of your week? If you could do your clinical time over again this week, what would you do over? What are your goals for next week? How did you feel getting that emotional component into it? How did you feel about clinical this week?' Those are always enlightening to me."

This nurse educator expresses a common concern of nurse educators: that students will be so focused on skills as tasks that they will ignore the judgment and thinking required to perform skills safely, or to see the bigger picture of the patient's clinical situation.

Pestolesi, along other nurse educators in programs we visited, helps students see the bigger picture. She and others evoke a world of practice in the classroom. They used pedagogical approaches that offered a contrast to teaching methods all too familiar to many students, where the teacher names and categorizes signs and symptoms in abstract generalized cases. In this paradigm case, we have tried to show how situated teaching helps students develop a sense of salience, clinical imagination, and clinical reasoning. In the next part, we turn to Lisa Day, another paradigm-case teacher, who helps her students integrate the three apprenticeships in ways that help them also develop their clinical imagination.

PART THREE

INTEGRATIVE TEACHING FOR CLINICAL IMAGINATION

If you see something in clinical and then study it in class, or study it in class and see it in clinical . . . it's just burned into your brain—what's going on, what's happening—and you never forget it.

As classroom observations and student survey responses consistently revealed, all too often students do not have the experience this student describes; nursing education separates acquisition of knowledge in the sciences, social sciences, and humanities in the classroom from experiential learning in clinical situations. Students are bewildered and dismayed at the marked contrast between the rich and effective learning experience of the clinical situation and the passive pedagogy of the nursing classroom.

Nursing educators must ask themselves how current classroom pedagogies help students prepare for nursing practice. Although memorizing the most general aspects of clinical conditions may help students see commonalities between patients, students then must make a significant effort to interpret how a categorization scheme or taxonomy translates into actual assessments and interventions in clinical situations, and to incorporate into those assessments and interventions for a particular patient's experience and concerns. The classification systems alone do not suggest how the student will use the information to care for patients and their families in the hospital, home, or community. Students are left to figure out the relevance of classifications of signs, symptoms, and interventions for meeting and caring for patients and clients in particular situations.

In the face of an ever-increasing amount of information to cover in the classroom, fewer faculty to teach the courses, and the growing press of students who want to become nurses, approaching the classroom with a packed outline and hundreds of slides may seem like an efficient practice. However, as Eraut (1994) points out, the kind of deliberative processes that professional practice demands cannot be developed solely through mastery of procedural or abstract information: "They [professionals] require unique combinations of propositional knowledge, situational knowledge and professional judgment. In most situations, there will not be a single correct answer, nor a guaranteed road to success; and even when there is a unique solution it will have to be recognized as such by discriminations which cannot be programmed in advance" (p. 112). Typically, professionals work in situations where there is uncertainty about outcomes, guidance from theory is only partially helpful, the context offers relevant but often insufficient information, there is limited time for deliberation, there is a strong tendency to follow accustomed patterns of thinking, and other professionals may be consulted or involved. To begin to develop the integrative thinking that professionals draw on in complex practice, nursing students need to acquire knowledge in a way that relates directly to the skilled know-how and ethical comportment they are developing in clinical situations, and to acquire knowledge in ways that allow them to imagine situations and rehearse for them.

Consider, for example, the approach of a classroom instructor who uses mapping rather than catalogues. As one of her former students explained, "She would lay down a pathophysiology issue or a problem. We had to identify the problem, prioritize our care and communicate the multi-disciplines that would be involved in that care and map out, from the pathophysiology to the meds, to the interdisciplines and back. And that was in second semester.... It changed how I approached all the disciplines in school as a student and it even changed my approach in study." Moreover, the student said, "It changed my personal practice and what I do as a licensed nurse."

Asking students to draw on their clinical experience in the classroom helps them imagine how they will use the information. Engaging them in extended simulations of clinical practice, such as case studies or simulated cases in a skills lab, is a means of integrating knowledge, skilled know-how, and ethical comportment, but it also helps develop their clinical imagination and sense of salience. One classroom teacher, for example, asks students to consider how they would react in complex situations, such as a case where a patient is in shock and the physician orders Propranolol: "I just leave it at that.... Is this correct or is it not correct? Well it's not correct, this is an emergency, the patient's in shock and tachycardia. How are you going to handle it? I like those discussions. It's not only about how you would care for the patient but what would happen if you were ... in a situation where not only were things ... wrong, but it fell on your shoulders. I have plenty of real examples. I don't have to make these things up." This kind of example places the student in a specific situation and requires situated thinking about action.

This instructor's students have an opportunity to use knowledge as they consider how and why they would act in a situation where there are clinical threats and dangers to the patient. Other uses of cases focus on the patient's concerns and coping during an illness trajectory. There is no list that could begin to cover the range of situations classroom teachers can use to simulate the open-ended situations nurses face daily. Nor is there a finite list of situations the aspiring professional can anticipate; the practitioner can only develop an imagination for practice in a broad and varied array of clinical situations.

The paradigm case of Lisa Day, a classroom and clinical instructor at the University of California, San Francisco,* illustrates that it is possible to effectively integrate knowledge and practice in the classroom by both mining and anticipating student clinical experiences. Day demonstrates an innovative and effective approach that could do much to decrease the overload of content in nursing curricula.

---

*Lisa Day is a member of our research team, but because she was a central teacher in the Master's Entry Program at the University of California, San Francisco, she recused herself as a researcher for this site visit, which was our first. She was chosen, by her colleagues, as a teacher to observe because she teaches a pivotal class at UCSF.

7

PARADIGM CASE

LISA DAY, CLASSROOM AND
CLINICAL INSTRUCTOR

Bird watching is my metaphor for teaching nursing. . . . I use slides of birds and point out the field marks on a bird, where you might see it, why it's so beautiful, and what it does in its life. And that's what I try to do with the acute care experience.

LISA DAY'S YEARS of bird watching have yielded a depth of knowledge that enables her to identify birds first by sound and then by sight. She describes the novice birder "trying to match what you see in the pictures to what you see in the field, and saying, 'Well, its head is red, but it's not really that red. And I don't see this little mark over here that's in the picture, so I don't think that's what it is'" and "that agonizing process . . . of becoming the expert, the point where you see it and you know what it is." No longer is identification "a matter of adding up the pieces, it's just, 'That's what it is.'"

Day knows birds in their own habitat, not as a series of analytical markers of identifying features. Similarly, she believes the goal of nursing to be understanding the patient in context, as a whole person with a life, a person who is responding to physiological challenges and illness. "The response from the birder is to put it on your list, but nursing requires a much more complex response." With the intent to help students develop the clinical imagination for nursing's "complex response," Day engages her students in a learning experience that, she believes, will help them give excellent, state-of-the-art nursing care.

She believes that the complex response that is high-quality nursing care can be effectively developed in both classroom and clinical situations, by deeply connecting the two. Through unfolding cases—ongoing clinical stories—Day, who teaches master's entry students, engages the students in today's patient's unfolding clinical situation; the process of problem solving directly related to the patient's situation is the classroom context for learning the science and skills of care.

She makes it clear to her students that she cannot teach them everything they need to know for practice—an impossible task. Instead, she models for them an approach to practice that places concerns about a patient, family, or community at the center of their attention. Her questions guide students toward integrating what they have learned in other classes and clinical situations and toward developing a sense of salience: grasping the nature of a clinical situation and recognizing what about it is more and less important. She is also teaching her students to be curious and effective clinical learners in the classroom and in their clinical assignments.

Combining questions, discussion, lecture, and graphic illustration, Day guides the students through a patient's clinical scenario over several class periods. As students and teacher reason together about how to respond to changes in the patient's condition, she models clinical imagination and reasoning and encourages the student to flex these skills. Day encourages her students to use evidence, always keeping in front of them the goal of doing what "needs to be done" for the well-being of the patient, including working with the collaborative team that is managing the patient and making a case to physicians for any medical interventions or changes.

Moreover, Day helps her students develop clinical imagination and acquire knowledge through the context of their emerging practice. Although she is a midcareer clinician who has been teaching for about seven years, she continues to volunteer for clinical shifts in the intensive care unit to keep up her clinical skills; the cases she uses most often come from her students' current clinical assignments. As she explains, "I try to make everything that we do in class relate to this particular patient. And this opens the discussion for other particular patients that they've seen and taken care of. If that doesn't happen naturally, I'll mention something about our case-study patient and how she responded to that intervention. Usually a student will say, 'Well, the patient I had who had this didn't respond in that way.' And then we can open a discussion: 'How did that patient differ from this one?' 'What sort of differences might you see?'"

Day also teaches some of her students in the clinical setting: "I have a group of eight students that I supervise directly, and I'm backup oversight for another seven at our site here. I know which patients they've been working with for the last week. When I'm in class, I can say, 'You had a patient that was similar to this. Tell us about that.' Or 'Your patient wasn't quite like this; how did she differ?'"

Noting that nurses need to develop appropriate responses to patient concerns and clinical conditions, Day explains that she seeks to help her students extend their imaginative reach: "Being able to evaluate your patients and how they present physically and anticipating the next step in their care—I think that's very important." To that end, as she makes use of comparisons between the patient presented in class and the students' current patients, she brings clinical experience directly into play, making the classroom a source for acquiring and using knowledge, rather than a place where science and nursing knowledge are taught abstractly. The students learn in order to understand the patient's situation and plan care. In doing so, they develop clinical imagination.

In short, Day's approach to classroom teaching, connecting clinical realities to classroom material, gives students a chance to imaginatively rehearse for practice. This is the kind of teaching that students who responded to the Carnegie-NSNA survey found mostly lacking in their schools.

Mrs. G.

In an amphitheater class, thirty-five students in Day's advanced medical-surgical nursing are looking at pictures from her bird-watching trip to the Sacramento Valley. She uses the photos to create a moment of relaxation before they begin their discussion about Mrs. G., a critically ill patient who is in intensive care. During the preceding class, Day introduced Mrs. G., a forty-five-year-old woman admitted to the hospital with a diagnosis of pneumonia and later found to be HIV positive. Now Mrs. G. is showing signs of sepsis.

On a large piece of paper, Day displays the questions that will focus the discussion for the entire class period:

- What are your concerns about this patient?
- What is the cause of the concern?
- What information do you need?
- What are you going to do about it?
- What is Mrs. G. experiencing?

Using these questions as a scaffold, Day leads the students through the process of collectively thinking aloud about Mrs. G.'s clinical situation, always guided by the goal, as she says, "to do well by the patient."

Throughout the class period, Day uses Mrs. G.'s evolving condition to explain the complex pathophysiology of sepsis, engaging the students in considering the implications of the patient's changing vital signs and laboratory results, such as blood gasses and the trend of white blood cell counts. She articulates those aspects of the case that, as she says, "nursing owns" while also pointing out how the health care team works together to care for the patient. Although the classroom discussion is an exploration of clinical implications, she frequently returns to what Mrs. G. is experiencing in the midst of increasing signs of septic shock and respiratory distress, thus always focusing the students' attention on the patient. With the goal of helping her students learn to both see and think like a nurse, Day engages them in and guides them through unfolding case study—a simulation of care, enlarging their clinical vision and imagination through experiential learning. Lisa Day is a calm and well-grounded teacher. Her students seem to be engaged because of the import of what she is teaching and the students' sense of confidence that she is a knowledgeable teacher as well as an astute listener. Sitting in the classroom, we observed Day and her students think out loud as they reasoned through the case while it changed over time. It is clear in the class that Day knows and respects her students' rich backgrounds as she invites them to contribute to the discussion.

Multiple Teaching Strategies

Day is an active classroom teacher. Throughout the discussion, she moves toward students, smiles, and makes eye contact, assuring them that she is a curious and respectful listener as they wrestle with the details of the case. Her patience, attention to detail, and mastery of the subject assuage the students' anxiety about grasping the complexities of sepsis. Her confidence gives students the sense that they will understand the process before the class is over. In fact, they do. Her deft use of multiple teaching strategies and examples gives the students different ways to understand the case, in effect more than one access point for understanding.

Lecture and Slides

In marked contrast to her counterparts in other nursing classrooms, for Day lecture and technology are just two among many pedagogical tools. For example, in the course of the class she incorporates a lecture on physiology. Saying "Sepsis is a big diagnosis," Day gives a comprehensive description of the physiologic changes that are occurring, using Power-Point to display pictures and diagrams and an overhead projector to show the feedback loops between aspects of the sepsis-associated physiological and biochemical cascades. Over the course of her explanation, Day used three diagrams to demonstrate interrelated aspects of sepsis. Later, when she moves to what is happening with Mrs. G. at a cellular level, she engages the students in solving a complex puzzle about multiple organ dysfunction; using PowerPoint slides that illustrate the process but do not label signs and symptoms, she asks the students to identify or match the symptoms from the case with a diagram of the systemic physiological events of sepsis.

In explaining how she uses lectures and slides, Day says nursing students need to know anatomy and physiology, but knowing them in the abstract is not sufficient for knowledgeable, effective care of a patient. For example, in describing another unfolding case of a patient with a transsphenoidal approach to pituitary surgery, "I use the picture of the transsphenoidal approach and they look at the anatomy and figure it out." She explains: "Some students have seen transsphenoidal surgery patients, post op. They haven't seen the surgeries, so I have pictures of how the probe works and what the entry point is. It's either through the nose or through the palate." The pictures are opportunities to ask the students to imagine "what if?"

As Day asks the students what the risks are, she points out, "'You can see the skull anatomy and where the pituitary sits; why is that approach a good one? But then, what are the risks? You go through this sinus and through the bone, through the dura.' Every time I do that, some student comes up with, 'Oh, cerebral spinal fluid leakage . . .' we talk about what you need to look for then, in terms of the clinical signs of that." Day comments, "I really enjoy that much more than lecturing. For the most part, I use pictures, not words, on the slides, to demonstrate what's happening with the patient."

It is important to note that although Day uses slides to illustrate concepts the case brings forward (for example, a diagram of endotracheal intubation, a diagram of the sepsis cascade), she does not use photographs or films of a patient or family; nor does she use a mannequin. She is aware that her reliance on student imagination is risky; not all the students have seen a patient in respiratory distress. However, by drawing on descriptions from students who have seen similar patient situations and filling in with accounts from her own practice, Day is able to bring students into the patient care experience authentically.

Dialogue and Questioning

Chief among Day's pedagogical strategies is dialogue and questioning, a familiar strategy from clinical instruction. As comments during interviews with students and responses on the Carnegie-NSNA survey consistently revealed, dialogue and questioning are the teaching strategies students most value in their clinical instructors. "During the clinicals, [the instructors] approach you and ask you questions: 'What's going on with this patient? What do you need to do next?' I found that that was incredibly helpful," explained one student. As another student commented, "It engages me . . . because she kind of leads . . . not tells you but gives you enough of a guide and asks, 'Are you thinking about this?' And then she gives you a little bit and then that will get your mind going."

Within the frame of her guiding questions, Day uses questions to invite the students into the process of clinical reasoning. As Day prompts students to make connections with past lectures as well as their clinical and other experiences, she asks follow-through questions, making sure that students know how to interpret a sign or symptom in a patient's situation. Consequently, she frequently asks "So what?" questions. She also guides the students in framing the questions that will help shape their practice as nurses: as she responds to the students' questions, she points out why one might be a "good" question or a "not-so-relevant question at this point" and then returns to the case study, always explaining the physiological basis for the answers.

Day's use of questions in her classroom about the patient and his or her experience in a clinical situation allows her students to rehearse how they think, see, or act in *that* situation. As she uses the unfolding case study, she asks students to join in a simulation of a clinical situation, where they can imagine and rehearse their reactions to an unfolding, changing situation. She asks the students to imagine aloud how they might see, think, and act as nurses in the situation. Her students work as a group, thus pooling their knowledge and skills of clinical imagination.

Day's students attribute their growth to her skilled use of questioning. As one student explained, "She presents us with a case study, she mimics what you would see in an acute care setting and then she'll question you: 'What do you see here? What's concerning you? What steps would you take? How would you address this? What things are critical to you at the moment?'"

Another student added, "We have to draw upon what we learned in the first quarter in order to answer those questions, in addition to what we're learning now . . . and our own clinical experiences."

Staging

Day also stages the material for her students. As the material becomes more difficult, she encourages the students, saying, "Step through the process and then we will go back and go over the main points." Repeatedly she backs up to go over points that the students do not understand. She also introduces complex material in familiar terms and then presents the technical vocabulary once they grasp the concepts. For example, when her goal is to help the students grasp the influence of large and small vessels on blood pressure, she starts at a broad, conceptual level, drawing on simple language, such as "the bad stuff" and "big vessels clamp down," as well as vernacular clinical practice language such as "the big vessels" for "aorta" and "vena cava." Likewise, Day uses vivid word pictures to describe the unfolding physiological events. She also clearly identifies "take home" messages.

Mining Student Experience

When asked how she coordinates what she is teaching with what the students are currently experiencing in their clinical assignments, Day maintains that using the unfolding case allows her students to mine their own clinical experiences: "Just giving them a patient situation to start off the conversation is helpful to get them thinking about what they've seen in their clinical."

Day also looks beyond her students' current clinical experience and draws on their prior life experiences. Most of her students are embarking on nursing as a second career, and some have worked in health-related careers prior to coming into nursing; she draws heavily on their prior experience. Knowing that her students have a baccalaureate degree and experience in other fields, Day seeks connections between the cases and the students' backgrounds, thus bringing the students' past knowledge or even expertise to bear on their current clinical experience.

She has great respect for her students' academic and experiential backgrounds and knows about her students' past and current clinical experiences. "I could talk about my students forever because I just think they're so interesting," she says. They also have a wide range of academic preparation. Noting that the eighty or so master's entry students are usually selected from among approximately five hundred applicants, chosen after careful screening and interviews, she says—and her students agree—that she "treats students like the graduate students they are."

She describes the range of student backgrounds: "They've had all sorts of other experiences, and some of them are direct health care experiences," such as women's health, or caring for persons who are HIV positive or with AIDS. "One student in my clinical group was an emergency medical technician in New York City; she's had some crisis intervention experience in health care ... [there are] others who have worked for Planned Parenthood and a few others who have been in the Peace Corps."

Day thus recognizes that some students, because of past experience in community or primary health care, may know more about clinical situations than she does:

> I'm an acute care clinician. I've lived in the hospital forever, and this is where I practice. This is the practice that I know. When I talk about patients who are hospitalized, I don't have a lot of feedback from the group because they're learning. This is the stuff that they're here to learn. But when I open the discussion about anything in primary care issues or health screening, a lot of them can contribute to that discussion. We go back and forth between what they know and can teach each other and what they're here for us to provide for them. For example, I'll say, "Here's this woman who has cervical cancer, and these were her risk factors. Now she's in the hospital for a total hysterectomy. How are you going to take care of her after that surgery?" Next week I lead the class in a discussion about HIV and AIDS, and I know there are students who have worked in clinics, so I know they're going to have a lot to contribute. I'm going to draw on that. I almost depend on it now because I don't really know the outpatient treatment. I know what happens when a patient is admitted and we know about their history and how it affects my plan of care for their hospitalization.

Using Knowledge

Day has just explained to the students how things can go wrong at a cellular level. Now she gives the students breaking information: Mrs. G. has new lab reports and vital signs to interpret, and new interventions (such as 100 percent oxygen by nonrebreather mask) have to be instituted. The discussion turns to treating the infection and transferring the patient to the ICU. Day reports that Mrs. G. "looks sucky," and she asks the students, "Why does she have edema?"

Mrs. G.'s evolving condition and attendant interventions now demand that the students draw on their knowledge of science and medicine. The students begin to sense that they are solving a mystery. Some important information seems to be missing. Then one of the students asks what the arterial blood gas (ABG) shows. "Great question," Day says, and reveals ABG results for Mrs. G. She asks the students to interpret this new piece of information: "I know one of you is thinking about anaerobic metabolism and lactic acidosis," she says, looking at a student who is interested in these subjects. She then returns to the diagram of the sepsis process and relates the new details relevant to the pathophysiology. She continues on the ABG, indicating the important diagnostic implications of the trend in Mrs. G.'s vital signs.

Day says, "Step back: Is Mrs. G. stable?" There is palpable tension about the case. Clearly, Mrs. G. is in respiratory distress and her clinical condition is deteriorating. Her body is working hard to restore physiologic stability. Then Days says, "We don't make any decisions on our own. We are part of a team. We will make a case." She summarizes all the evidence that the patient is in respiratory distress and headed for probable respiratory crisis and then says, "Here are the facts, including new lab results of lower ABGs even after the 100 percent O_2 rebreathing mask intervention. Here is our assessment. Take this to the resident. The data should be sufficient to get immediate action—in this case, endotracheal intubation. You want to make sure that all measures have been tried to prevent the need for intubation first, but in Mrs. G.'s case they have been done, and there is no doubt that intubation as soon as possible is the right intervention." Day tells the students that if they do not get immediate action from the resident on duty, they must immediately go up the well-established chain of command for a second opinion.

When Mrs. G. is intubated, Day shows a picture of an endotracheal tube and leaves it on the screen while passing around a real endotracheal tube to the class, asking the students to look at it and figure out what problems might occur as a result of intubation. She then covers a number of clinical issues related to endotracheal tubes, pointing out specific nursing concerns when critically ill patients are intubated: preventing pneumonia and tissue breakdown, and promoting comfort and support. She asks, "What are the nursing interventions that can be put into place?" She uses evidence-based medicine and nursing and refers to the American Association of Critical Care Nurses (AACN) recommendations for prevention of ventilator-associated pneumonia. Day brings up from the Internet an adult respiratory distress syndrome protocol from NIH's Heart, Blood and Lung Institute (NHLBI ARDS Network, 2004) that gives a good explanation of why a patient like Mrs. G. requires low-volume ventilation. She explains "barotraumas," tissue damage from air pressure, giving a name to the condition after explaining it. In discussing pneumonia, Day identifies mouth care as an aspect of care that "nurses own." She emphasizes that since nurses instituted routine interventions such as oral suctioning and elevation of the head of the bed, the incidence of ventilator-associated pneumonia has decreased. By bringing in this and the ARDS information, she also models for the students the integration of evidence-based medical and nursing care as an expectation for practice.

As Day talks about Mrs. G.'s experience of air hunger, and then her decreased alertness, the students are responding as if they are her concerned and effective nurses. When she explains that the pulmonary arterial line is introduced, she uses pictures of the catheter and pictures of waveforms created by it as it is threaded through the two valves in the right heart and into the pulmonary artery (PA), where it will "wedge," temporarily occluding blood flow. "I'm glad you feel the tension. If you don't see how the wedge reading reflects left heart filling pressure, let it sink in, just trust," Day says. Demonstrating that the seriousness of the situation calls for urgent and focused attention, she engages the students in problem solving around issues of the PA line and wedge pressure measurements, giving feedback about their responses.

At this point in the case, she suspends the process. Next week, the class will learn about what impact the interventions that were made today will have on Mrs. G.

Developing a Complex Response

Simulation of care for one patient whom students come to know over several classes engages students in thinking about how they might react as nurses. The case of Mrs. G., for example, involved Day's students in imagining how they would respond to the increasingly grave situation. As the students imagine caring for Mrs. G., they integrate their understanding of the relevant science with skilled know-how and ethical comportment in order to respond to the situation appropriately, for the good of the patient. They engage in productive thinking, or in Eraut's terms *using knowledge* appropriately to care for their patients. Knowledge use, as Eraut points out, is distinct from knowledge acquisition, or even direct application of technical knowledge; knowledge use requires productive thinking and innovation in particular situations (Eraut, 1994).

Although the students we spoke with after class mentioned that they understood they had much more to learn about septic shock, they valued the experience of being asked to exercise a clinical mode of thinking about a particular patient across time. Stereotypes and overgeneralizations seldom occur with this approach. The specificity of the patient's experience demands good clinical judgment and an understanding of the clinical situation and the patient's plight. The students are encouraged to consider the patient with respect and dignity, something that is difficult to achieve with composite and artificial cases. "In this class," the students told us, "our imaginations are drawn into the story, a compelling clinical situation where we are asked to respond as *nurses*."

8

DEVELOPING A CLINICAL IMAGINATION

IN OUR INTERVIEWS and from the Carnegie-NSNA survey responses, students reported that on the whole their experience of learning in the classroom did not develop their clinical imagination. As a student responding to the survey noted with dismay, "I don't feel you get enough practice and guidance in the classroom that best fits how the settings will be in the clinical setting." Our classroom observations corroborated the students' views that clinical integration is missing in most nursing classrooms.

"I feel that much of what we learn in the classroom," wrote another student on the Carnegie-NSNA survey, "has no direct implication with the day-to-day clinical setting. I wish there was more hands-on [practice] in the classroom setting [with] how to deal with a client and more pathophysiology in the clinical setting." Another student pinpointed difficulties students and teachers face in the classroom when trying to teach and learn nursing practice: "The classroom tries to inform us of the skills and knowledge we will need in the clinical experience, but the reality of the clinical experience is hard to obtain or explain in a classroom setting. There is a great difference between what is taught in the classroom and 'real-world' practice."

In contrast, Lisa Day's students point out that her classroom simulation of an unfolding case and her clinical questions for students integrate what they learn in the classroom with what they learn in clinical settings—"real-world practice." Developing students' clinical imagination helps them both recognize significant changes in a patient's condition and make a persuasive argument for a change in therapy. Day creates opportunities for students to rehearse using clinical reasoning in transition, following patient changes that require them to think in a number of ways in order to respond appropriately. Similarly, she uses the students' involvement in cases to extend their imagination about practice to working with the health care team. For her students, the clinical learning thus flows back and forth from the hospital and other clinical situations to the classroom. In large part, this happens because she considers aspects of practice that the students must prepare for, such as learning to stay open and learning to make a case.

Learning to Stay Open

For Day, teaching critical care and medical-surgical nursing in the hospital setting cannot be separated into technical mastery plus clinical judgment and ethical comportment. The three are intertwined. Technical mastery and knowledge are necessary but not sufficient for becoming a good nurse; the nurse's therapeutic responses must be generated by the patient's concerns and clinical situation. In other words, the nurse must stay open to changes in the patient's responses over time and recognize the clinical implications of any trends in the patient's vital signs, urinary output, or other relevant aspects of patient changes.

In her classroom, Day uses the unfolding case to drive home the import of attention to changes in a patient's condition over time, a key learning point for nursing practice. Because it is the nurse who spends the most time with the patient, a crucial part of nursing practice is detecting patient changes and then adjusting nursing care accordingly, which may include alerting physicians in order to prompt adjustments or changes in medical treatments. It is important that nurses avoid ritualized responses and routines so they are always open to the possibility that the situation may call for something different.

Clinical teachers must constantly help students master the skilled know-how of practice while at the same time encourage them to stay open to what is unknown, always ready to have their assumptions turned around. Students need to learn how to assess the patient's immediate history to account for changes in the patient's current condition and at the same time reason across real-time transitions as the patient's condition and concerns continue to evolve. Thus nurse educators put a great deal of effort into teaching students the importance of ongoing assessment over time with attention to what is different now, and clinical faculty spend time instilling a disposition for being open, as exemplified in this exchange:

> I brought the case to the student: "So what would you do next? This patient isn't fitting the profile. The patient isn't going along like you

expected. How can you revise this plan?" And that's the thinking piece, because we don't want to give students blueprints but have them adjust their care to go along with the person's current developmental stage, to go along with the cultural status of the patient, what they normally eat. So we teach the student to think in a lot of different directions instead of putting things in boxes most of the time. "This is the patient, this happens, what do you do next?" And they *can't* look at their notes and memorize how to answer the question. They really have to do some thinking. How can they adjust their plan and how they can deal with the fact that what they prepared for on Monday night is not at all what they're going to do on Tuesday?

By drawing the student's attention to the shortcomings of a plan made the night before, the teacher in this example helped her student learn how to stay open and think in a changing situation.

Day brings the same focus on vigilant assessment and openness into the classroom: "And then we bring the patient into the unit [and say], 'These are your first assessment findings. What else do you need to know?' They come up with all kinds of other things. I purposely leave some things out of the assessment for them to find. They come up with all kinds of other stuff that's missing that I didn't really even think of or maybe isn't essential information right at this moment, but definitely is going to make a contribution to what you know about this patient."

The Power of Context

Day's approach to classroom teaching suggests how contextualizing practice helps students stay open: focus on the patient and respond appropriately to a patient's specific needs and concerns. Likewise, her goal in clinical teaching is that students focus on the patient rather than the "procedure of the day." As students learn technical skills such as placement of a nasogastric (NG) tube, they also learn to form appropriate responses to the particular patient.

Day writes an ethics column, "Current Controversies," for the *American Journal of Critical Care*. In this excerpt of a column Day wrote with Minnie Woods, a beginning nursing student working on a general surgical unit, Day illustrates the focus on the patient that she stresses with her students in the classroom as well as in clinical. Woods writes:

> I was assigned to Mrs. R. She was diagnosed with a small bowel obstruction secondary to pancreatic cancer. During report they said that Mrs. R. had been overwhelmed by nausea throughout the previous

night and that she needed to have an NG tube placed but that she was refusing it. My first thought was, "Thank God she's refusing it," because I knew that it would be my responsibility to insert it.

Since I started nursing school, I've been completely terrified of NG tubes and the whole idea of inserting them. I remember looking through our nursing skills book my first quarter and thinking that having such a big tube put through your nose down to your stomach seemed like one of the most terrible things I could possibly imagine, never mind actually doing it to another human being.

I sat in report that morning hoping that I was off the hook because Mrs. R. didn't want an NG tube anyway. As soon as report was over, I checked in with the staff nurse I was working with that day. I said, "So it sounds like Mrs. R. is pretty nauseated and miserable but she's refusing the NG tube." "That's right," my nurse said, "so you better get in there and convince her that she really needs it." I knew she was right, but I was completely dreading the whole experience.

I was already pretty familiar with Mrs. R.'s history and condition because I did lots of research the night before. When I walked in the room, Mrs. R. could barely open her eyes. She was completely overcome with nausea and was hesitant to even move. Her abdomen was really distended. Suddenly, here was this woman that I was taking care of who really needed some relief from this tremendous discomfort. I sat down and talked to Mrs. R. about the NG tube and why she didn't want it. She was scared, of course, and wondered if it was necessary. I explained how the procedure would work, that I would do it myself with the supervision of the staff nurse, and that once we began to suction out all the fluid that was building up in her stomach she would start to feel some relief from the nausea. She agreed to go ahead with the procedure.

Putting the NG tube in wasn't even that remarkable. It happened just like in the nursing skills books. We connected the NG tube to suction and in the first hour drained 700 mL from Mrs. R.'s stomach. About 1,450 mL total after 8 hours.

That whole day was a real turning point for me. Before that, I was completely focused on myself—my own fears, anxieties, incompetence, and disgust. But when I met Mrs. R. and really understood her suffering, the NG tube was transformed from this thing I was terrified of to this thing that could alleviate Mrs. R.'s misery. A couple of hours later, after a lot of suction, Mrs. R. wasn't feeling nauseated anymore. When I went into her room to check on her she said, "Thank you so much for convincing me to get this tube put in. I feel so much better" [Day, 2005, p. 436].

As Day comments, Woods's experience is a story of transition from a focus on technical skills to a focus on what the patient needs:

> The story points to the power of knowing and taking seriously what is at stake in any patient care situation. Had the student taken up the opportunity to place the NG tube as simply a chance to practice and perfect her own skills, given her aversion to the idea of placing the tube, she might have continued to avoid the procedure by deferring to a thin notion of patient autonomy. Instead, the student's confrontation with the patient's suffering, and realization of the patient's need for the tube, went beyond her technical knowledge of the tube's purpose, beyond her technical knowledge of the procedure, and beyond familiarity with the patient's condition gained from the medical record. The student's response to what she experienced firsthand and rightly perceived as the patient's need helped to avert the clinical emergency of a perforated bowel or trauma associated with vomiting. The response also averted the ethical dilemma that arises when a patient refuses a simple, ultimately comforting and potentially life-prolonging intervention [Day, 2005, p. 436].

The students in her classroom are likewise engaged in ethical responses. Day's use of the unfolding case brings into the classroom the experience of relating to the patient's concerns and experiences and to the team in the clinical arena, always driving home the message that good nursing care is about the patient, not the nurse, and skills of engagement with the patient's concerns and clinical needs are essential to deploying the most appropriate knowledge and skilled know-how.

For this reason, Day brings the practice of nursing into the classroom. She structures the interactions in class so that the students become participating nurses consulting with Day as a clinical nurse specialist on the acute management of a patient. The students must pay attention to the salience of the patient's situation and imagine appropriate and well-timed interventions in response to the patient's quickly moving trajectory. The students in the class we observed left with a sense of what is salient in Mrs. G.'s situation, and how to prioritize the actions they should take.

Learning to Make a Case

In the classroom, Day emphasizes that students are part of a health care team, with nurses responsible for some tasks and doctors others. During the class discussion of Mrs. G., for example, she used a set of questions to bring the physician into the picture: "So then the patient progresses, you get a set of physicians' orders. What do you think is important to implement right away? What's missing from this? What are you going to call the doc and ask for if the doctor forgot maybe this or that? Or, what are you going to question in the set of orders? What raises a question for you?"

The ability to speak to other members of the health care team about changing a patient's treatment or care is an essential nursing skill, and both students and faculty refer to the student's first call to a physician to suggest a change in care as a milestone. As one clinical instructor explained, "They can't take phone orders, so we'll get on the phone with them, but I always have [the student] call [the physician], and very often it's their first experience with calling a physician about a patient and I get the deer-in-the-headlights look when I tell them, 'You've got to call the doctor.'"

One student noted that the experience of making a case is coming late in her program: "In the very beginning we didn't have the skills to know who [to] call, or for that matter ... [the] feeling that you are competent to have a conversation with a doctor on a phone about your patient. But now they're pulling all that in this last semester so we have to and are prepared when we graduate and we're on our own."

With the exception of a few nursing educators, however, we found very little formal attention to teaching students how to communicate with physicians regarding changes in patients, concerns they have with a patient, or recommended changes in therapies. Although many faculty acknowledge the importance of being able to make a case, they typically do not use the classroom as a place to teach students how to construct an argument, marshal and organize evidence, and present the case. Several instructors discussed the need for students to learn to be concise, present a problem, and frame a solution, but few offer students opportunities to practice skillfully making a case for an actual patient. Yet the classroom and skills or simulation lab can be a place to prepare for and reflect on experiential learning in the student's clinical assignment, such as making a case to a health care provider or making an error, or successfully noticing significant changes in a patient. Even if a student nurse understands fully the scientific evidence for what is happening to a patient, comes up with a solution to change the care for that patient, and is concise in the recitation of facts, all this may not be enough to capture the complexity and nuance of a patient's situation. Student nurses have an advantage if they learn a frequently used case presentation strategy such as SBAR, a communication tool. The acronym SBAR stands for *Situation*, a brief statement of the problem; *Background* relevant for the situation at hand; *Assessment*, a summary of what the clinician believes is the underlying cause and its severity; and *Recommendation*, what is needed to resolve the situation (Pope, Rodzen, & Spross, 2008; "SBAR Technique for Communication," 2007; Carroll, 2007). The SBAR tool is useful for making a clear and concise case and in reducing communication barriers.

Putting the Pieces Together: Integrative Teaching and Learning

With every unfolding case, Day asks her students to pull together the information they would need before calling the physician and discusses with them how to go up the chain of command if necessary. Her questions—What is the patient experiencing? What are your concerns about this patient? What is the cause of the concern? What information do you need? What are you going to do about it?—give her students a framework for making a case. She explains that she and the students use these questions as they talk about calling the physician and making a case. She might lead with, "What and how are you going to make your case that you need this order changed to something else?" That discussion leads to a conversation about planning the care: "So what's your priority nursing diagnosis? What are the goals that relate to that priority, and then what are the interventions that you might plan?" After Day runs through this process for two or three nursing diagnoses related to the case patient's situation, she will announce a change in the patient's condition: "Now, what are you going to do? What's the priority now that this has happened?"

For her students, the process of making a case in the context of planning care demands that they use their knowledge of physiological and practical ramifications as well as clinical reasoning. Coaching students on how to alert physicians to significant changes in a patient's clinical condition or the need for changes in therapy helps them develop clinical reasoning and clinical judgment as well as skills of communication.

Learning to make a case helps students develop strong communication skills. Most often the nurse is giving a firsthand assessment to the physician who is not on site; without benefit of seeing the patient, the distant physician has to be able to imagine the changes in the patient and assess the changes in vital signs and lab results over time. In all clinical areas, but particularly in neonatal and pediatric units, the challenge of making a case, from a nurse's perspective, is to present clear descriptive information about the patient's condition, such as color, energy level, alertness, and level of consciousness, in addition to the objective lab results and vital signs. If the nurse is vague or cannot give concrete comparisons between how the patient was earlier and is now, the physician may find it difficult to believe a change has occurred in the patient's condition or imagine the described changes.

Rehearsing the process of making a case supports students in understanding an important difference in perspective that nurses and physicians have on a given intervention. Each has the best interests of the patient in mind. For nurses, the error of making an unnecessary call is insignificant compared to the error of failing to call about a significant change in the patient's condition; for the physician, no action is usually safer than risky action. Students need to understand that this difference in perspective frequently leads to conflict between doctors and nurses, especially when they fail to appreciate the other's perspective, but the dialogue that occurs in making their respective cases usually results in better decisions by both parties on behalf of the patient.

Rehearsing for Practice

Well rehearsed in calling the physician and making a case, Day's clinical students thus describe calling a physician as if phoning a colleague. Even so, she continues to use questions to help clinical students pull together the necessary information before making the call. As another nurse educator describes this essential clinical instruction:

> We had an incident a day or two ago. . .this man was new. He had come in the night before, so nobody knew him that well. But he was just Dr. Jekyll and Mr. Hyde, one minute he would be as nice as he could be, and the next minute he was belligerent, kicking, and screaming. Then he would get weak and fall back. I had her just look at him objectively and asked her what the vital signs were. The vital signs were OK, but they seemed to change from 7:00, when we came in, to 9:00 or 10:00, when we started noticing this behavior. I said, "Well what do you think you ought to do?" She said, "Maybe I need to take some more vital signs". . .his oxygen saturation was 80 percent, so I said, "What should we do next?" "We need to put oxygen on him, but we can't do that without a doctor's order." "Go to the telephone and call the doctor and tell him what's going on." I was really proud of her.

Day and other nursing educators use questioning, either in situated role playing or situated coaching, to help students learn how to effectively make a case. As one faculty member told us, "We do scenarios with them, we do some role playing. . .[we ask them] 'What do you do when you call?

What information do you have to have?'" Another teacher described her approach, pretending to be the doctor and saying to the student, "Tell me what you're going to say, whatever it might be. It might be something as simple as the temperature is up and we don't have Tylenol ordered." "They're always nervous to call," she observed. "They're afraid they're going to get fussed at. . . . And they'll say, 'I'm a student and I'm calling to let you know I've been looking over Mr. Smith today and he has a fever and we don't have any Tylenol order, can we . . . ?' I always tell them, give them a solution to whatever your problem is, if you can: 'Can we have some Tylenol?'"

Other nursing educators who give their students opportunities to rehearse making a case emphasized the need to teach the student to frame the problem and present a solution for the physician. One instructor uses an example from midwifery that she also uses in her undergraduate teaching: "Nurse midwifery has to occur in a situation that allows for consultation with a physician consultant, and there are two ways to consult: one is to go present the information and ask the question; the other is to present the information with a plan." She encourages her students to say, "This is what's going on; this is my plan" instead of asking, "What do I do now?" She does so, she explained, "By constantly asking them 'What's going on? What's your plan?' By *plan* I mean plan of care: What's the next test you're going to request an order for, or what other interventions or noninterventions are you going to choose? And how do you support that based on physiology and pathophysiology, based on policy of the hospital, medical legal issues?"

Students identified simulations in the skills labs as being extremely useful for preparing them for clinical assignments such as making a case, and a recent study on student learning points to simulation as a promising strategy (Brannan, White, & Bezanson, 2008). However, students and educators alike noted that simulation equipment is underused, and teachers noted a lack of faculty development resources and time for creating effective simulation exercises. We note that simulation offers opportunities for teaching and learning about interprofessional communication and teamwork. Planned simulations can, for example, present opportunities for students to formulate and articulate patient concerns to other members of the health care team, as well as to learn about common misunderstandings that occur in the clinical setting and more effective ways of communicating. Students from different health care professions can use simulation exercises to learn about their common perspectives and the particular contributions of the various team members.

Learning a Common Language

Some nursing educators stress that students must learn to use appropriate language as well as practice being organized and concise when they phone a doctor. Nurses, observed one faculty member, "are the ones who are with the patients twenty-four, seven. So they need to have all the pathophysiology, the pharmacology, because they are the ones who are there and then they need to transmit that information to the doctors whenever it changes." However, she noted, "I really feel this divide between the doctors and the nurses and all these different groups; you have to speak the same language in order to get respect and in order to get them to listen to you. If you're on the phone calling them in the middle of the night, they don't want to hear you mumbling. They want to know exactly what you're thinking, and they're going to take you seriously." "They need to learn to talk directly," explained another instructor:

> I force [my undergraduates] to write five-page papers—to do a case and write it in a five-page paper. They'll say, "There's no way, I can't get it all in there." I say back to them, "Concise, succinct, well organized communication is respect for communication. Your colleagues won't have ten pages to be able to listen to you. You have to learn how to communicate concisely to be able to be a respected colleague." And that changes it for them ... [they say] "This is a skill I have to learn...." I teach them the most basic common language because I want them to be able to talk and participate.

What Uncertainty Reveals

To make a case, the nurse must be able to structure the information in order to persuade, not simply inform. Thus, being able to draw on the material of the nursing classroom is essential to marshaling evidence. For the student who has been asked to memorize catalogues of information rather than learn the knowledge in meaningful context, the cognitive leap is great. Nursing educators told us that they understand the students' uncertainty as "lack of confidence" and encourage them to become more assertive. In fact, as interviews and survey responses consistently revealed, the students are uncertain about their knowledge of physiology, pharmacology, and other areas of nursing science. The students know that their grasp of the relevant knowledge is weak, which means that simply being more assertive is not enough.

The students' uncertainty underscores the need for nursing education to use more effective pedagogy in the nursing classroom. As one faculty member commented, "Many students see class and clinical as two separate courses. While most have integrated much of the content by the end of the quarter, we still see a good number of students [who] seem to know how to do patient care in clinical but cannot explain why they do what they do, other possible options, consequences of actions, or specifics of evaluation needs. Students still have great difficulty going beyond the objective health care data to see the person behind the 'patient.'"

In the next chapter, we turn to specific ways to make the nursing classroom a more effective place for integrative teaching and learning.

9

CONNECTING CLASSROOM AND CLINICAL THROUGH INTEGRATIVE TEACHING AND LEARNING

Classroom and clinical content often seem disjointed from one another. Information learned in clinical does not generally appear on classroom tests. Clinical experience draws on social interaction skills not taught in class.

THIS STUDENT COMMENT from the Carnegie-NSNA survey is representative of students' observations about the divide between the nursing classroom and the clinical experience. Faculty and students at many schools make a distinct separation between theory and practice; separate learning objectives suggest that thinking, problem solving, and interpersonal processes are discrete activities. Yet the nurse must integrate all of them in practice, and do so fluidly and appropriately for the safety and well-being of the patient. By connecting the classroom material and clinical learning through unfolding cases, Day gives students a safe space to learn what to pay attention to, and to try out ideas for real patient care.

Another student responding to the Carnegie-NSNA survey reported her difficulty in trying to integrate her learning: "While the program does require clinical write-ups, which require applying classroom content, I feel like I'm on my own in integrating the information we're taught. I spend quite a bit of time in independent study trying to fill in holes and gaps in my education that are revealed as I struggle in the clinical setting."

As the student comment that opens Part Three suggests, connections between the classroom and the clinical setting go a long way toward helping students grasp the knowledge on which their patients will depend. Students note that when their clinical instructor also teaches the course, the course objectives and content benefit from "direct clinical setting examples": "The teacher will say, 'Remember, we talked about this subject in class...here is a prime example of that lecture in the clinical setting.'" Yet students also recognize when their program makes a concerted effort to draw classroom and clinical together; as one student observed, "They try to...give us bits and pieces and work altogether and make sure that they're all on the same track and trying to complement what we're learning in one class to another. So it's all tied together." However, "Until faculty integrates content, we cannot expect students to do so," asserted one nursing educator.

Of course, dual clinical and classroom teaching assignments facilitate integration. "Classroom faculty [in our institution]," one faculty member explained on the Carnegie-NLN survey, "are also the clinical faculty augmented by some adjunct faculty. We know exactly where the students are contentwise and select learning experiences accordingly." "It's helpful when you are the classroom teacher going into clinicals," said another faculty member. "Sometimes it is easier to relate to theory in clinical because the client is right in [the student's] face." Another teacher noted that in clinical she tries to place her students "with patients who have the disease process we are currently discussing in class." Day notes, "If the students are struggling in clinical, I can return to the classroom and clarify content, perhaps present it in a different way."

Despite the hard work of teaching in the classroom and practicing in the clinical setting, the reward is being able to bring currency about practice to their students, as one faculty member notes: "Because I work sixteen hours a month in a local hospital plus donate time to a local free medical clinic, I can integrate a lot of true and timely situations into my teaching. I also am not only lecturing about the problems in health care and the nursing shortage; I am living them out."

Even when the faculty have separate classroom and clinical assignments, it is possible to bridge the divide. One faculty member described her program's policy: "Clinical experiences emphasize content taught in the classroom. Each adjunct clinical faculty is given the classroom content and appropriate postconference topics to mesh with classroom content. Some clinical experiences are also timed to match content in the classroom." One school's clinical and classroom faculty meet every other week to discuss classroom and clinical integration and the clinical learning, including difficulties of particular students. This program was unique among the nine we visited. Clinical faculty receive extensive orientation and instruction prior to and during teaching. In addition, clinical faculty are reimbursed for time spent in the biweekly team meeting and required in-service classes on clinical instruction. This school makes a concerted effort to bring the clinical and classroom teachers together to share the responsibility for students' integrative learning. The teachers' development is highly valued by the service sector because it prepares staff nurses for teaching within the health care setting.

Where such policies are not in effect, however, as the clinical teacher's comments suggest, "Those who teach in clinical settings and those in classrooms need to know what each is doing. . . . All clinical instructors have access to classroom content via textbook and Web supplement." Using such information, she brings the classroom into postclinical conferences: "[I say] 'Last week in class, you discussed the problem X that your patient has. How does your patient compare with what you learned in class?' Or, 'Your patient had X. You will be talking about this next week in class. Think about your patient again during class.'" She continued: "Not all faculty do this. Some [clinical] faculty [members] aren't even aware of what topics were covered in classes the previous week. I created a one-page grid of all topics in all classes by the week for myself and have shared it with other faculty. Seeing the information on one page is very helpful when making clinical assignments and knowing what skills or information students have or have not had in class."

Another instructor pointed out that "clinical instructors meet to discuss clinical learning and also discuss clinical situations by e-mail during the weeks of clinical experience." This comment illustrates that the flow of information needs to go from clinical to classroom and vice versa. School policies can help teachers better integrate classroom and clinical teaching. For example, one faculty member spoke with admiration about how the clinical faculty in her program receives "a weekly run-down of the kind of things that are going on in each course." She pointed to the example of students learning about communication and cultural differences, and how knowing about this can be very important in clinical situations, noting that students "can think not only about the fact that they are learning about burn injuries but they're also learning how to communicate with a specific person [across cultural boundaries and languages] about their injuries and concerns."

Despite such avowed commitment to integration, all too often nursing education is approached as if it has two discrete elements. As a student comment on the Carnegie-NSNA survey noted, "It is as if the classroom content was a different program."

Integrative Teaching, Integrative Learning

Integrative teaching—teaching that not only integrates the classroom and clinical but helps students integrate knowledge, skilled know-how, and ethical comportment—prepares students to function in clinical situations. Students rehearse clinical situations of practice in order to learn how to use their communication skills and in-depth knowledge of pathophysiology and pharmacology, and attend to patient well-being and other salient patient and family concerns. Integrative teaching fully recognizes the limits of trying to make everything explicit and instead focuses on helping students understand the situation sufficiently to draw on their relevant knowledge or search for any information they may not have. To that end, integrative teaching explicitly connects knowledge acquisition, knowledge use, clinical imagination, and ethical comportment. Questions such as those Day asks stretch the student's ability to recognize the nature of the clinical situation and respond appropriately: What is the patient experiencing? What are your nursing concerns? What information do you need? What are you going to do about it?

Locus of Responsibility

We found differing opinions on who is responsible for integration. We found teachers who saw it as their and their institution's responsibility to help students integrate clinical and classroom learning, as well as humanities, social sciences, psychology, pathophysiology, and nursing. One faculty member describes her senior-level course:

> I tell the students. . .that this is the opportunity to integrate everything [they've] learned in the last three and three quarter years, and I really let them function very autonomously and then probe them very carefully about how they manage new patients. Not just the patient but looking at the developmental stage of the child, looking at the family, looking at discharge planning and then also, what's going on with them in the hospital at the same time. And I teach them to begin to be patient care managers. And then along with that, being part of a team, being a nurse: "What does that mean? How do you interact with others on the unit?"

Yet many teachers consider integration of classroom and clinical to be up to the student, as one educator remarked: "Students are expected to apply theoretical knowledge in the clinical setting, and build on the clinical practice as the curriculum progresses." Some teachers pointed to the student, rather than the approach to teaching: "Students do not seem to be able to transfer or apply material from general education (anatomy and physiology, growth and development, microbiology, etc.) into the clinical setting." We believe, however, that making such a distinction between knowledge acquisition and knowledge use—thinking that students just "apply" their knowledge as if it were mere transfer of information—overlooks the productive thinking and clinical imagination required for using knowledge in a practice discipline. In contrast, integrative teaching helps students learn to simultaneously draw on knowledge, experience, and ethical concerns in practice situations. A nursing educator's description of her program's approach in postclinical conference suggests how integration can be effected:

> [We] ask them...to present a case that they saw that day. And they take turns, and they were expected to present the physiologic changes that were occurring: "Describe what the pathophysiology was that might have been occurring. Talk about the social implications for that family as to what was going on. Talk about policy: Why did she get a C-section, or why didn't she get a C-section? How did the things that were done as part of her care or the neonatal care influence the outcome?" They were forced to go back to all their core courses and pull it [knowledge learned] into their recent clinical experience on some level.

The questions the students wrestle with in postclinical conference cross many domains: health policy, pathophysiology, and the care of the family, to name a few. By helping students integrate their fresh clinical experiences with past learning, these teachers encourage the habit of reflecting on practice for the sake practice improvement.

Pedagogies of Integration

The very strength of pedagogical approaches in the clinical setting is itself a persuasive argument for intentional integration of knowledge, clinical reasoning, and skilled know-how and ethical comportment across the nursing curriculum. For example, Dewey's mandate (1933) to reflect on experience formed the rationale for pre- and postclinical conferences and deliberations, which are almost universal in nursing education. Reflective journals, narrative accounts of clinical experiential learning, are common clinical assignments for students in addition to care plans made in advance of their clinical assignments, and revised on the basis of changes in the patient.

Indeed, among the professions in the Carnegie Foundation studies, nursing education in the clinical setting stands out as having a uniquely strong emphasis on developing and mining experiential learning through reflection and narrative understanding of transitions in the patient's condition and care over time. Nurse educators typically guide nursing students to discover aspects of clinical patient care that they did not anticipate in their planning, and students are also expected to improve their practice the second day of a clinical assignment as a result of reflecting on their experience. Students exchange hard-won experiential clinical lessons with their classmates and consequently enlarge their collective understanding of nursing practice. Students and faculty prod, encourage, and compliment one another on their difficult and rewarding clinical learning. We found that clinical groups were highly interactive and effective learning communities. Many clinical instructors do an outstanding job of creating a climate of safety and trust, so that students can safely explore their mistakes as well as their accomplishments in clinical practice in their learning communities. Many teachers are also forthcoming about their own lack of knowledge, the need to keep learning, and their past clinical mistakes. Nursing students typically share a culture of actively disclosing their experiential learning—even their mistakes—with their classmates. Day, like Pestolesi, teaches in both classroom and clinical settings and tries to integrate the two arenas. The dialogue between clinical and classroom and vice versa is pervasive in Day's teaching.

In the classroom, Day gives her students a forum in which they can imagine and rehearse how they might act in a clinical setting. Students are invited to form a vision for practice, and to focus, as the example of Minnie Woods illustrates, on developing the most appropriate responses to patient situations. Teachers who contextualize science and other relevant domains of nursing knowledge learn to formulate the most important clinical concerns, set priorities for action, and communicate effectively with the health care team.

Although the shared learning experience is familiar in the clinical setting, it may not be an immediately comfortable approach in the classroom. The class we observed Day teach has much in common with the narrative approach. Diekelmann and Smythe describe the focus of narrative pedagogy as a shared learning experience:

> [The teacher] also decenters herself as a teacher when she asks the question, "How are we to think about treating diabetic neuropathy?"—a question with more than one answer. She joins the students on an exploration that does not tell, but rather invites thinking and further

questioning. [This] kind of questioning resists a focus on "an answer" and on the teacher as expert. The teacher does not walk out of such a class knowing that a long list of content has been covered. Rather [the teacher] emerges from a shared experience of learning with her students, sensing their eagerness to continue the quest to understand more, and knowing she has equipped them for the ongoing learning process [Diekelmann & Smythe, 2004, p. 344].

Day asks many questions for which there is more than one answer and gives a sense of sharing with her students the quest to deliver the best care to Mrs. G. as she progresses toward septic shock. Day uses no list of content to be covered. Instead, she lets students grapple with the content questions as they come up in the course of the case: Why is Mrs. G. edematous? What signs of organ failure is Mrs. G. exhibiting? What are the risks of endotracheal intubation? What can we do to help Mrs. G. tolerate low-volume mechanical ventilation? How can we help her cope with her anxiety? Day uses her clinical expertise and actively guides students to see clinical situations as nurses. There may be more than one answer to her question, but there are also wrong answers, and she makes it clear to students when they are paying attention to the wrong things. A wrong answer is a teaching opportunity to keep students focused on what is most salient. She addresses with a direct response a question from a student that would steer the discussion into an area that is not relevant to the patient's care at this moment: "That's a good question, but I'm not worried about that right now." The students and Day work together as a team to provide the best care for a particular patient.

PROBLEM-BASED LEARNING.   The pedagogy of unfolding cases is most similar to problem-based learning (often referred to as PBL). Yuan, Williams, and Fan describe PBL as "a student-centered approach to learning which enables the students to work cooperatively in small groups for seeking solutions to situations/problems" (2008, p. 657). Whereas the key feature of the unfolding case study is that it is an ongoing, changing situation in which the nurse's focus of attention and priorities change, students participating in a PBL exercise typically receive one unchanging scenario, a clinical situation involving a patient, to work through in a small group. As Day's students do with her unfolding cases, the PBL students grapple with the information and its implications for care as they work together to identify the patient's problems and form a plan to address them. To address the problem successfully, the students are expected to draw on past learning to identify gaps in their knowledge, and search out information. With their evidence, each small group discusses and decides on a plan and then presents and defends the plan in a larger group discussion (Williams, 2001). The unfolding case study encourages students to engage in situated cognition and reasoning across time to develop appropriate interventions as the patient's condition changes. According to Williams:

> Learners exposed to PBL as an instructional methodology acquire knowledge and skill in nursing by encountering real practice situations as the initial stimulus for their learning rather than as a culminating activity. Learners grapple with the complexities of the situations, search for connections across disciplines, and use existing and newly acquired knowledge to generate outcomes. When they have identified possible outcomes they present, justify and debate each possibility, searching for the best possible outcome. Learners collaborate with classmates to refine and enhance their knowledge and skills. They build substantial knowledge and skill bases within the discipline of nursing and across other disciplines through reflection and critical reflection [Williams, 2001, pp. 27–34].

SIMULATION. Unfolding cases, PBL, and other similarly engaging pedagogies offer a means to integrate the kind of learning that today's nurses need for practice. Day's use of unfolding case studies in the classroom is also a form of simulation that asks students to enter into an active clinical discussion in which something is at stake for a simulated patient. Simulation has been used in medical and nursing education for many years, and with the recent rise in nursing school enrollment coupled with limited clinical placements interest in simulation as an adjunct to clinical teaching and learning in nursing has exploded (Landeen & Jeffries, 2008). There are many types of simulation, and they may or may not include a high-tech or high-fidelity component. There are benefits to the highest-fidelity mannequins, which can imitate a patient's physiologic as well as human responses to disease (Seropian, Brown, Gavilanes, & Driggers, 2004a). Seropian and colleagues also point out the danger of purchasing expensive simulation equipment without developing a solid plan for its use in teaching and learning. Some nurse educators fear that simulation mannequins will be used only for practicing psychomotor skills, when the technology is more suitable for higher-level thinking and problem-solving exercises (Seropian, Brown, Gavilanes, & Driggers, 2004b).

As Landeen and Jeffries (2008) note in their editorial introducing a special issue of the *Journal of Nursing Education* on simulation, more research is needed on its limits and opportunities. There are some promising approaches, as Wong et al. (2008) illustrate in their discussion of problem-based learning used in conjunction with simulation. Another report on simulation from Thompson and Bonnel (2008) illustrates the possibilities simulation offers for teaching more than skills. Another area worthy of further attention is interpersonal communication. Despite advanced technological tools to simulate patient communication, as used at this time, we wonder, however, whether simulations may be less valuable for learning skills of interpersonal communication with patients and recognizing the nature of the interpersonal concerns of the patient than for making clinical interventions. We worry that the use of patient mannequins does not bring into play the full range of human interaction in human encounters, such as nonverbal cues or psychological withdrawal. The experience is less realistic, less ambiguous than real clinical situations. The use of patient actors is more realistic. In the end, students need to experience risks, threats, and opportunities for care and patient well-being in order to improve their situated thinking and communication, or their ability to think and communicate while in a situation. Such a high-level communication skill requires reflection on practice in both simulated and real situations.

As a form of simulation, the unfolding case study takes on a narrative structure that relies on the student's imagination to fill out the picture. The role of a narrative unfolding case needs to be studied in terms of its effectiveness as a source of clinical imagination and rehearsal for likely clinical situations for the learner. As we noted earlier, although Day uses images to illustrate concepts that the case brings forward (such as a diagram of endotracheal intubation or of the sepsis cascade), she uses neither photographs nor films of patients, nor any kind of mannequin for demonstration. The reliance on student imagination is risky; not all the students have seen a patient in respiratory distress. However, by drawing on descriptions from students who have seen similar patient situations and filling in with stories from her own practice, Day is able to bring students into the patient care experience authentically.

PART FOUR

TEACHING
FOR MORAL
IMAGINATION

We are privy to these very, very critical moments in people's lives. Especially, because a lot of us are younger, most of us have never experienced any of these feelings in our lives before. All of a sudden you are in a room with somebody who's just been told that they may only have a couple more weeks to live, or that the treatment they're getting isn't working, or that they have the diagnosis that they've been fearing. For us to be there standing by and experiencing that suddenly puts us in a very intimate relation with them ... we've been there with them when they've experienced that.

THE ABILITY TO quickly form effective relationships and act with compassion is necessary to good nursing practice, as this student's observation suggests. Seriously ill children; women in labor; patients recovering from open-heart, abdominal, or orthopedic surgery; patients whose communication is compromised by illness or injury; mentally ill patients in escalating anger episodes; elderly patients with cognitive impairment; family, friends, and others close to the patient who are trying to convey the patient's concerns—all these and countless others rely on the nurse's moral imagination as well as her knowledge and skilled know-how.

Another student explained, "You kind of get caught up in all the tasks and we all want to do tasks, but you also have to remember that there's a person at the end of the bed and that's just as important as putting in an IV." As this student nurse understands, in any situation or setting, whether caring for patients through critical illnesses, recovery, or rehabilitation or helping people prevent illness and promote their health and well-being, good nursing practice requires knowledge, skill, and moral imagination.

To learn to focus on the "person at the end of the bed" while expertly inserting the IV, the student must form new habits of thought and action and relinquish old habits and perceptions. Some nurse educators call this process *formation* and *re-formation*. Others call it *socialization*, acquisition of *professional values*, or development of *professional identity*. We suggest the term *formation* because it denotes development of perceptual abilities, the ability to draw on knowledge and skilled know-how, and a way of being and acting in practice and in the world. Formation occurs over time with the transformation from the well-meaning layperson to the nurse who is prepared to respond with respect and skill to people who are vulnerable or suffering. Formation occurs when students acquire and learn to use knowledge and when changes occur in their perceptual capacities to act with skilled know-how. With knowledge and experiential learning, students develop notions of good from their practice that transform their understanding of nursing's social contract to care for vulnerable patients.

Although teaching and coaching for ethical comportment are strengths of nurse educators, it is important for nurse educators and students to recognize that the formation of dispositions, skilled know-how, and perceptual skills occur in *every* aspect of a nursing student's education. Classroom and clinical teaching need enrichment and integration, so that knowledge use becomes as important as knowledge acquisition. Teaching for clinical and moral imagination is essential to any professional education, but especially important to nursing education since nursing practice is relatively unstructured in range and kinds of practice situations. Students are formed by all they do, all they read, all they perceive and interpret, and in all models of practice—not only in the context of what they think or know intellectually, but also in terms of their taken-for-granted assumptions and expectations.

As noted earlier formation occurs through the formal curricula; in implicit curricular agendas or hidden curricula, and in all learning arenas. No profession has greater responsibility with more vulnerable populations than do nurses. For example, the nurse who makes her patients unnecessarily worried, frightened, or dependent through lack of communication, relational skill, self-knowledge, or ethical insight can cause great patient-family harm. In contrast, the nurse who is astute about the treatment demands, patient concerns, and coping challenges can significantly impact patient safety and well-being.

Teaching and learning ethical comportment in interpersonal and relational skills requires thoughtfulness, good curricular, and pedagogical development and planning. For example, nursing educators expect students to prepare for their clinical assignments by reading and researching their patients' clinical conditions and therapies. At the end of the clinical day, educators commonly use clinical debriefing seminars to guide students in reflecting on their clinical experience. During these seminars, teachers ask students how they might improve on their day's practice, a strategy that emphasizes the expectation that they will develop a self-improving practice and pursue lifelong learning. The expectation that students will prepare for clinical assignments and participate in seminars where they reflect on their experiences should be preserved and improved.

As noted in Chapter Four, we like Mohrmann's use of the metaphor of dance (2006) as a metaphor for formation because it is relational and changes appropriately and knowingly according to the context, partner, and music (that is, the possibilities in the situation). Formation occurs as a result of knowledge, skilled know-how, and ethical comportment learned in many concrete situations over time.

Students learn how to use knowledge, develop skilled know-how, and internalize ethical comportment—all for the good of the patient—when they are continuously made aware of the "the person at the end of the bed," ceaselessly asked to focus on what works and what does not work in specific clinical situations, and constantly given opportunities to feel the risks of "falling short" (Kerdeman, 2004). Thus, although abstract principles and technical skills are necessary for orienting and alerting the learner to appropriate regions of concern and competency, they alone do not prepare the learner for the complexities of practice. Through engagement with clinical problems and particular patients and patient populations, students broaden their moral imagination, just as they broaden it by literature, nursing knowledge, bioethics, and the ethics of care and responsibility.

The classroom can also be an evocative place for students to develop moral imagination. To illustrate, we present the paradigm case of Sarah Shannon, who teaches ethics to baccalaureate and master's entry nursing students at a large research university, the University of Washington in Seattle, and who conducts research on ethics and consults as an ethicist.

PARADIGM CASE

SARAH SHANNON, NURSE ETHICIST

I want to develop keels for them . . . they come oftentimes with pretty
flat-bottom boats and the trouble with a flat-bottom boat is, when the
wind blows, you just scatter across the water. And the wind blows this
way, you scatter back across the water.

KNOWING HER STUDENTS will need to act ethically in situations fraught
with conflict and confusion, Sarah Shannon explicitly focuses her teaching
on formation. Using questions and dialogue, she challenges her students
to thoroughly understand the clinical situation and facts of each situation. She engages them in a lively dialogue that helps them uncover their
assumptions. There are high stakes in the teaching of ethics, and Shannon
is clear that she wants her students to avoid the dangerous ethical shoals
of complete relativism and subjectivism. She wants her students, as she
says, to develop moral keels and self-understanding while at the same time
respecting the values and perspectives of others—to become nurses who
are inclusive and nonjudgmental.

Her accounts of teaching constantly point to her ultimate goal of formation. Although she has immediate content goals, they are always in
the service of shaping nurses who will think and act ethically, who will
respect the diversity of values and the ambiguity inherent in clinical practice, who will remember that right action in nursing is always about the
patient.

I want them to come out of the course with a clear sense of their professional values. I talk a lot about [the fact] that professional values are
the social contract we have with patients. They're what every patient

can expect when a nurse walks in the room, whether that nurse is young or old, male or female, black, white, regardless of their ethnicity, regardless of their religion, regardless of anything. It's your social contract. For example, your personal value might be that you really like openness. Your professional value is that you adhere to confidentiality. That's the contract with the patient.

Shannon, who has been teaching her ethics course for eight years, has an active and ongoing research and consulting career as an ethicist. Her passion for teaching ethics is evident: "I love teaching this course. . . . A lot of people struggle with how to teach this content . . . this shocks me when I find out that often it's not a popular class with students in other programs, that they actually hate the class and find it boring. I'm dumbfounded. . . . [The students] want to do my readings: they're fascinating."

Her grasp of the subject is comprehensive and seasoned by her research practice and ethics and consultation practice. She admits the advantage she has in her teaching because of her immersion in and expertise about the subject she is teaching: "Everything I do is ethics: I teach ethics, my research is on ethics, yesterday I spoke on ethics." However, she describes her development as a teacher as a difficult process. As a novice teacher, she tried to "cover everything." She recalls scrambling to cover the proliferating issues in ethics and her gradual shift to a more process-oriented approach:

> I would have this list of topics . . . I need to cover withdrawal of tube feeding, I need to cover stopping chemotherapy . . . I would just have lists and lists of all these issues. I packed the content in. What I've come around to is that I want them to learn a process that they can apply to another case. I also want them to learn what they don't know, which is the hardest thing to teach people. Not that I'm going to teach them what they don't know, but I want them to *own* what they don't know. So, I want them to look at a case and . . . be able to say, "Well, I don't know whether it's painful to die of dehydration. Gosh, you know, I have this initial reaction, but do I have any evidence for that?"

In paying attention to her experiences in the classroom and what her students were learning and what they were not, Shannon recognized that her most important responsibility is to teach her students how to think ethically about taking care of patients, and how to separate their personal feelings about patients from their professional responsibilities to them. Once students understand how to think about ethical problems, she believes, they can act in an ethically responsible way.

The Case

Shannon conducts each class as a dialogue about the cases and related articles the students read in advance. The class session we observed was early in the term, at the point where she establishes the basic framework she and the students will use for analysis throughout the term, Jonsen's fourfold ethical analysis structure (Jonsen, Siegler, & Winslade, 2002). In this particular class meeting, Shannon opened by asking the students to choose from among the cases they had read. They chose the internationally publicized Terry Schiavo case, with its attendant religious, political, and family controversies over withdrawal of fluids and nutrition from a young woman in a persistent vegetative state.

Shannon sets the classroom up so that students face each other. After she outlines the case, a student asks a question. Turning to the other students, Shannon asks, "What do you all think about that?" She uses that invitation to comment as a way of starting a conversation among the students. As the students discuss the case and their fellow student's question, she does not intervene, letting them "dig their holes." From time to time she says, "We'll come back to this and talk about why this is an important distinction."

Then she steps in and moves the discussion from the case to a more systematic approach, saying, "In ethical decision making, all of these questions come up. I want to give you a framework for thinking about these cases." She outlines the Jonsen framework for clinical ethical decision making (Jonsen et al., 2002), telling them, "You are going to want to become *facile* in this." Then she again walks the students through an analysis of the Schiavo case, this time using the Jonsen model.

Knowing the facts helps families make decisions, and Shannon tells her students they must be clear about the clinical issues because they have a moral responsibility to get it right before they talk to patients and families. Thus they must always be clear about what is fact and what is their private opinion, whether informed or uninformed. She tells them too that before offering a treatment option to patients and families they must always ask themselves whether the option *makes sense* clinically in the situation at hand.

Shannon now draws in the relevant science and philosophy central to the case. She asks, "How do you define *consciousness*?" After assuring the students ("I want to give you permission to say 'I don't know'"), she explains the pathophysiology of persistent vegetative state (PVS) and coma as well as the respective treatment options. About treatment options, she says, "We have to be clear about these. I can't emphasize this enough."

When she then engages the students in a discussion about the implications of the various aspects of PVS and coma, she uses a series of guiding questions: "If we agree she's in a PVS, does she have the capacity for pain?" and "If she doesn't feel pain, what does *comfort care* mean?" When she asks, "Why would it be painful to die of dehydration?" she offers the hospice nurse's maxim, "Better to die dry."

Once the students are clear about the clinical issues they are dealing with and the treatment options available, she moves on to consider the role of the patient's preferences in ethical decision making. She discusses the principle of autonomy, and how one considers the preferences of patients who are confused or unconscious, especially when there is contention among family members and providers about what the patient's preferences would have been. Next, she takes up quality-of-life issues, asking the students to consider what deficits the patient will have if treatment is pursued. Finally, she introduces the "contextual features" (Jonsen et al., 2002) of the case, telling the students sternly, "This is where we own our own biases." She lays out the conflicts between family members and providers in the Schiavo case, asks the students to consider who the primary beneficiary of treatment is, and discusses the underlying issues of justice, fairness, and fidelity.

Throughout the discussion, Shannon carefully keeps her views on the case in the background; instead, she draws out students' hidden biases as she helps them articulate their own views, their understanding of their role as professionals, and their responsibility to the patient and the family:

> I use the case and then say to them, "OK, now imagine this was you. How many of you would want X and how many of you wouldn't want it?" And then I say, "Look around. We don't have societal consensus on this. Thinking, caring, good people, educated people disagree with one another...." One of the reasons I use so much class discussion is that I want them to realize that while they may view themselves as pretty homogeneous... they are not, and it helps them to see... then I say, "Just imagine: You are privileged students. You're college educated. Right there, you're privileged.... Just imagine the diversity of opinion that occurs across America.... We don't have societal consensus on the Terry Schiavo cases." And so I try to emphasize to them, "So what's your role? To compassionately care for these people, to not pass judgment, certainly to not pass judgment, and treat them differently."

Shannon's strategy of laying out the case and allowing the students to wrestle with the issues before she enters the discussion as a provocateur is something she learned from one of her mentors, Thomas McCormick, an ethicist in the medical school at the University of Washington:

> What he does, and what I try to do, is to create this environment where people feel free to say what they want, what they're feeling, and when they say it, he very kindly helps them dig a hole. . . . But the trick is, you offer them a hand out. . . . And so, what I try to do is align myself with all positions, help them dig holes, because it's helpful for me to have the worse-case scenario. Oftentimes if a student has really dug into a hole, I not only offer them a hand out but I might go back to them at the end of the conversation and say just in the group . . . "What I just want to come back to is, what would *you* want?"

The "hand out" that Shannon offers her students is a framework for thinking about cases as a nurse and a language with which they can converse with their colleagues when they are working as nurses: "I jump right into applied clinical ethics." Although she does not teach normative ethics as a working framework, she does expose her students because "it is helping to teach them the norms . . . I don't want them to get out there and get stomped on when they try to engage in these conversations. So, part of teaching them [is teaching] the language of the principles [of normative ethics], even though there are more sophisticated ways of looking at ethics. I teach them the most basic shared common language because I want them to be able to talk and participate [in ethics conferences in practice]."

Her students commented on the efficacy of her approach. One student explained, "She respected us, plus she had this way . . . you were sure about something, and she had this way of making you see a whole other side to it. And suddenly you'd be scratching your head, saying, 'Well, maybe I wouldn't do that. What would I do?' And then she would guide us through the process of trying to understand the case." Another observed:

> She would pose a case, saying, "This is the scenario," and then she'd say, "So what would you do?" and somebody would say, "Well, I would do this, this is what I think I would do." Then she would question them and say, "Well, have you thought about this and what about that?" and then get other people's input. Other people would have different perspectives and she would get a lot of discussion going in the class and a lot of people did have differing opinions and different perspectives and she brought it out in a way that we weren't trying to kill each other and at the end of the class—we all left with good feelings about one another. I don't know how she did that sometimes because

there were some pretty varied opinions, but I never felt like, "Boy, what a stupid opinion."

Shannon ends each class by summing up. She describes the students' thinking processes and what they established as the facts of the case. She connects issues from the day's discussion to issues discussed in prior classes, and she notes particular issues that will come up again in other cases. Today, for example, she refers to the discussion of surrogate decision making from the previous week and then points to where this will lead in the next class.

Modeling Ethical Comportment

Shannon's classes seem to be fluid, guided by readings the students have done and the cases they select for class discussion. Each class unfolds as the dialogue that uncovers and clarifies students' values and beliefs. Yet she has a larger plan for the course. With a clear focus on the case and ethical issues at hand, she keeps the class discussion focused on the day's topic. Class discussions become more sophisticated as the class progresses. Ethical distinctions that students did not notice in earlier classes become clearer as the course progresses. Individual students' ethical stances also become clearer as the class progresses.

Thus, in contrast to courses or lectures that are assembled from standardized outlines or PowerPoint slides, Shannon's ethics course unwinds, like thread coming off a spool, with each class connected to the others behind it and ahead of it. She has a sense of the whole course over time and where these particular students are in relation to the whole and what she needs to do to get them to the next stage. To accomplish this, she must know the subject, know her students as thinkers and moral beings, and above all keep the patient at the center. (Shannon constantly says to her students, "It isn't about you, it's about the patient and the family. What you personally think doesn't matter. It's how you act professionally as a nurse that matters.") She is always thinking about ends and means, what she has to go back to, what she has to reframe because she sees that the students did not understand.

As she strives to teach her students how to think and function ethically and practically in the real world of nursing, she is firm about her expectations for their conduct as nurses, acting always on behalf of the good of the patient. She teaches students to do reflective, ethical thinking and expects her students to master the basic science, clinical knowledge, and skills necessary to care appropriately for their patients, making informed ethical decisions. The students understand that these are not arbitrarily high standards, for her purposes alone; they know that Shannon wants them to be exemplary nurses, and they learn the social contract of the profession. Above all, her focus is always on the kind of nurse she wants her students to be and the kind of moral agency she wants them to embody in a health care setting. She prepares her students to go into the clinical setting and function effectively as members of the health care team, able to make their case about ethically difficult clinical situations.

Accordingly, she continuously asks her students to consider the implications of what they are saying, to push themselves to more ethically grounded ways of thinking, to examine their biases and predispositions as well as the multiple perspectives of all the participants in the case. She demands clear thinking, or as she describes it, "recognizing when you've made assumptions and being willing to question those assumptions upstream, and then being willing to entertain multiple perspectives, embracing ambiguity. For me, it's a necessary part of moral imagination."

Shannon approaches teaching as an ethical practice shaped by her notions of what good nursing practice demands and what ethical care of patients requires. Her classes, usually around twenty students, become a moral community over the course of the class. Recognizing her important role in shaping her students, she demands of herself ongoing professional and personal growth. Because her approach depends on the students' responses to the case, she cannot completely lay out the class ahead of time. She does not present slides, for example. Things sometimes surprise her. When she sometimes misjudges the students' background, ability, or level of knowledge about nursing, she must figure out, on the spot, how to go back and revisit the content differently. She even uses her own mistakes to model ethical behavior: "It's a little scary. I go into every class and sometimes I trip and fall. When I blunder, give them the wrong information, I try to correct myself. So I model what you do when you blunder. If I think I've hurt somebody's feelings, I will deal with it in private, if that seems the right way, and I'll say to them, 'I'm sorry.' I try to model the kind of professional behavior I want them to take forward ... But it's risky."

Her course stands in stark contrast to many classes, where the subject matter is divided into discrete modules taught by rotating faculty members who may not adapt their lecture to the particular class. Shannon's approach considers that students must be prepared for the complex responses required in practice, and she understands that they will soon be called on to use knowledge, skilled know-how, and ethical comportment in the service of interpreting a dynamic, fluid clinical situation—for the good of the patient.

II

BEING A NURSE

FORMATION, AS NOTED EARLIER, occurs as students develop knowledge, skilled capacities, and insights into the notions of the good that are central to nursing practice. Thus it cannot be restricted to prespecified locations or even course objectives. In formation, personal and professional transformation are central. This chapter focuses primarily on experiential learning in clinical and informal learning settings.

Theories of socialization typically do not account for the profound development that many nursing students experience in sensory perception, skilled know-how, and capacities for engaging in relationships with patients and families. Nor do socialization theories adequately account for the sense of wholesale personal transformation that many nursing students describe—the point at which they feel as though they *are* nurses—and how participation in nursing practice creates a meaningful existence that, for many students, is markedly different from their life as lay persons or beginning students. The lay student moves from *acting* like a nurse to *being* a nurse.

As the example of Sarah Shannon's classroom suggests, learning in a practice discipline such as nursing requires more than socialization into prescribed roles and adoption of a prescribed set of beliefs. The process of formation—developing and using situated knowledge and skilled know-how, and learning ways of perceiving and acting ethically—is arduous. As Dunne (1997) observes, "A practice is not just a surface on which one can display instant virtuosity. It grounds one in a tradition that has been formed through an elaborate development and that exists at any juncture only in the dispositions (slowly and perhaps painfully acquired) of its recognized practitioners" (p. 378).

In both interviews and survey responses, advanced-level students and beginning nurses frequently described how their sense of mission, or call-ing, made it possible for them to withstand the rigors of learning for practice and gave them the courage to enter high-stakes situations, where the consequence of a mistake can be enormous. The students claim that this understanding of the significance of their work and their identifica-tion with nursing practice were what kept them focused through terrifying clinical situations, heavy or conflicting academic demands, and compet-ing family and work responsibilities—any of which might have led them to drop out. They cite classmates who were performing well but who did not identify themselves with the significance and relevance of nursing practice and consequently chose to drop out of the program. Students describe finding what Taylor (2007) calls a "moral source": "Coming to clarity about [our motivations] why we are doing this can help identify and neutralize other extraneous motives...which may muddy action and lead us away from our goals. And it [moral sources] will characteristically also inspire us to strengthen our resolve. A motivation which has this kind of potential to empower I want to call a 'moral source'" (p. 673).

Doing, Knowing, Being

Nurses enact their knowledge of the natural and human sciences, technol-ogy, and ethics and are able to transform this knowledge into the capacity to perceive and act in a given situation. Students' descriptions of how they learn in clinical situations to perceive, think, and act like a nurse are consistent with accounts of learning to *use* knowledge (Eraut, 1994; Lave & Wenger, 1991). Bourdieu (1990) uses the term *habitus* to describe the situated, tacit knowledge of inhabitants of a culture or practitioners of a complex practice. As the practitioner develops a habitus, incorpo-rating taken-for-granted meanings, knowledge, and skill, it recedes to the background, becoming part of a complex web of the practitioner's assumptions, expectations, understanding, and skilled capacities. As a result of developing new perceptual capacities, a sense of salience, and skilled know-how, a habitus is formed and available to the practitioner. The practitioner develops the capacity to become attuned to each familiar situation (Benner et al., 1999; Lave & Wenger, 1991).

As nursing students develop habitus, instructors formally recognize them as nurses. An instructor in a BSN program observed: "In the second semester of the junior year, everyone begins typically calling the students 'Nurse.' You might ask them to do a patient assessment, and at first, they say, 'I'll go get the nurse and she will do it.' 'Wait a minute, you *are* the nurse.' And I think it's that realization, coupled with either [sic] the complexity of the pathophysiology and the medications that the patient is on, and also recognizing, 'I have to be organized. I just can't run around in circles any more. I have to focus myself, get organized, have a plan.'"

As students progress from caring for one or two patients to larger patient assignments, the situation shifts dramatically; complex, busy clinical assignments call for learning new ways of organizing and planning. The students must learn "styles of practice" (Merleau-Ponty, 1962) that attend to the demands and priorities of patients in diverse situations. Even though styles of practice, or performance, bear a family resemblance to one another, the student must learn to respond to the salient clinical and human issues of each unique situation.

Style of practice is not limited to performing technical skills or learning to cope with inflicting discomfort on patients. Skillful and helpful ways of being with patients who are suffering vary according to the severity and intrusiveness of therapies, and on the patient's own coping responses. Although they may not use the term *formation*, many nurse educators deliberately foster the student's movement from a lay person's understanding of what nurses do to an insider's professional understanding of being a nurse and thinking like a nurse. Characteristic of this process is a shift in focus from mastering technique—producing replicable and predictable outcomes—to exercising flexible judgment and taking astute, context-dependent action in an underdetermined situation.

A faculty member describes how she encourages this shift from the start, even in skills lab:

> The skills lab really lays out a lot of those fundamental things for nursing, and that's what the students are totally focused on when they get there. They think if they can learn how to give a shot, they're a nurse. We explain to them that is not the be-all and end-all in nursing. I think a lot of lay people think nurses give shots and put in IVs and make beds . . . and these students are comparable to lay people when they first start. They don't always know what nursing is all about. So I think that's where we start to get the ball rolling . . . you have to spend a lot of time on those fundamental skills so that they become rote, and the students don't have to think step by step how to do a blood pressure and how to give a shot and how to put in a catheter, because then that frees them up for the higher-level skills . . . thinking and decision making and applying knowledge to taking care of patients. So, that's definitely a big piece of starting to help them think like a nurse. And we really do try to start to explain that to the students: "Yes, this is very important to your learning, but skills are a very small part of what nurses do."

Such messages in skills lab and elsewhere are important, but making the transformation to practice also depends on experiences that change the student's capacity to use and act on knowledge in a complex situation. The temptation is to reduce the notion of moral agency to a possession of skill and strategic capacities. However, strategic skillfulness and knowledge ignores the relational issues involved in good nursing care. The merely strategically skilled nurse would not need a good "bedside manner." However, the relationship between a patient and nurse depends on trust. Taylor (1985c) counters the attribution of strategic prowess as the essential characteristic of human agency with this: "Agents are beings for whom things matter, who are subjects of significance" (p. 104). By this he means that taking a stance on the kind of person one wants to be shapes human agency even though strategic powers and possibilities might permit disparate choices and actions.

Re-Forming the Senses

Nurses work daily with sights, sounds, odors, and tactile sensations that in other parts of their lives they might find repugnant. Whereas seasoned nurses and nurse educators often forget how or when they learned to cope with the sights, sounds, smells, and discomforts of patient care, student nurses new to the environment find it challenging to encounter bodily odors, for example, and the often-noxious odors of the hospital. Students must re-form their interpretation of bodily odors as common, not repugnant or even socially taboo. We noted that the important process of retraining the senses, so necessary for assessment and acceptance of patients in vulnerable circumstances, is rarely given significant attention in nursing education. It is easy to overlook something so subtle in a packed curriculum. However, by giving attention to students' reactions to the sensory challenges of nursing, educators and staff nurses can offer strategies for retraining the senses and also teach students strategies for using the senses in assessment.

Some educators do focus on the sensory. For example, one nurse educator who prepares new students for the sights, sounds, and smells they will encounter in clinical situations notes how it contributes to their transformation. She offered the example of preparing her students for the odors they will encounter when caring for a patient with a new colostomy:

> I'm talking with the sophomores about the smells. So yesterday, one
> of my students asked a question about tomorrow's patient assignment
> in postclinical conference, and I said, "This person is going to be

incontinent, they're going to sneeze, they may vomit. What are you going to do?" They all sat there. Then someone said, "I can't stand it when someone vomits." So I think it's this clinical world that's a major confrontation for them. And as a faculty member who takes them for the very first day, I literally walk across that bridge with them. And here we are, and they do such an incredible job. I'm going to cry, they do such an incredible job that by the fourth day they're nurses. They are different people.

Student nurses must also learn new ways to touch that comfort the patient while also producing important assessment data (Weiss, 1992). For example, a student might touch a patient in order to listen to heart sounds or palpate the abdomen. Touching patients in this new capacity requires that the student develop a professional demeanor and style of comportment that conveys concern and instills confidence in the patient while also demonstrating the student's technical competence. This is extremely difficult for most students, especially when they are not yet sure of what they are "palpating" or how the patient will respond to their touch.

For example, an educator in maternal-child nursing describes the difficulty students have when learning to feel the location and firmness of the fundus (upper portion of the uterus) after a woman has given birth:

Our students tend to be so frightened of checking the fundus and actually putting their hands on the patient, because it's the first time they've done an extensive assessment of a patient. They've done a history and physical on an elderly patient in a nursing home in the previous course and then, of course, practiced on each other. But as far as a patient in a hospital who's just had any kind of procedure or being around body fluids, this is their first experience with that. And so when they feel the fundus they say in postclinical conference, "I found it, I really touched the fundus, I couldn't believe I could really feel it," like they don't believe us when we tell them, "Of course you can feel it."

Re-Forming Social Sensibilities

Developing habitus and styles of performance enable the practitioner to be engaged with varying forms or degrees of involvement according to the situation. Students must quickly come to grips with the amount of suffering they will witness as nurses and the full extent of the manifestations of human illness and injury and their treatments. As one educator commented, "Even in pediatrics, students confront the difficulty of seeing kids who are badly injured or have multiple surgeries. A lot of students come in to be pediatric nurses and then they work with kids who are sick. And so they realize, 'This isn't going to be exactly what I thought it was going to be. I'm going to see some tough things' and it's hard. It's hard."

Not only must students learn to face people every day in situations and conditions that the lay person does not typically see; they must also learn to respond helpfully to people who have unusual or antisocial behavior. A nurse educator who teaches psychiatric nursing explains: "We deal in areas with patients that nobody else wants to know about too much. People don't want to talk about sexual areas; depression, drug and alcohol abuse in our society are hidden. And we're the ones who have to get in there and ask those questions. It's hard for the students to be able to talk with somebody who has schizophrenia or someone who's delusional or has a drug and alcohol problem that's pretty severe, so we role-model how to talk with patients."

As this educator points out, students face difficult work in re-forming how they relate to others, even down to the questions they might ask a patient. In effect, nursing students must learn to change the boundaries of their social access. For example, students develop relational attunement as they learn to read facial and bodily expressions in a given situation.

Sometimes the patient is compromised by dementia and difficult to meet as a person who has a history, likes, and dislikes. One student gave a moving account of caring for a confused elderly woman who thought the student was her own daughter. The student tried to correct the patient but gave in to the patient's recognition response when the student's corrections did not stick. The student gave the woman a bed bath, brushed her teeth, and brushed her hair while the woman continued to believe it was her own daughter providing the care. By meeting the patient as a person, she felt her care revealed the woman in a different light.

Re-Forming Skills of Personal Involvement

A student learning to insert a nasogastric tube will focus on the task, thinking out the steps of the procedure and preparing for the outflow of gastric juices. Yet, as Minnie Woods's experience related in Chapter Nine suggests, to incorporate fully the skills of the procedure into caring for the "person at the end of the bed" students must quickly progress from practical knowledge, or skilled know-how, to insight and understanding of the patient's fears, and how and why procedures are needed for the patient's recovery or comfort.

Student nurses talk readily about the interpersonal challenges they face in nursing. The process of learning some of the important lessons in the skills of involvement can be pleasantly surprising. A student nurse describes her initial pediatric experience:

> I like kids. I just don't want to take care of them. I don't like the crying and the screaming, the, "You're going to take your meds" and they're, like, "No!" And I just don't like the fighting. So I had a seven-year-old boy who had compartment syndrome. He had broken his arm earlier in the summer and now had an infection. They had to open the wound and it was horrible, and he was in a bed for weeks and weeks. He was three hours from home, and his mom could only come in for a couple of days out of the whole week, and so his grandmother was there sometimes and sometimes his aunt. He was just really, really miserable, the poor kid. He would get really agitated.
>
> Somehow I ended up bonding with him.... It had been raining for a week, and the sun came out. Being an idiot, I asked, "Have you been outside recently, have you looked out the window?" And he said, "No." (He could not see out the window and could not go outside.) So I asked, "What do you think you could see outside that window?" (I was trying to correct my mistake.) He started drawing, and that's how the window drawings started. I started drawing on the windows with dry-erase marker...and I would draw landscapes and I would ask him to imagine whatever he would see outside. It ranged from cowboys and Indians to army men in tents. I filled whole windows up with pictures for him.
>
> After that, any time I asked him to do anything, he would just say, "OK." I let him wrap my arm in a towel and pretend it was a cast so that he could do neuro[logical] checks on me. I started to actually enjoy pediatrics. That was dangerous!

In studies of skill acquisition, it was found that nurses who did not learn effective skills of involvement with the problem or situation at hand, or as it related to interpersonal relationships with patients, families, and team members, did not go on to become expert nurses (Benner et al., 1999; Benner, Tanner, & Chesla, 2009; Rubin, 2009). In our study, we noted that very often skillful involvement with the interpersonal aspects and the specific situation occur in direct patient care or are located in the hidden curriculum, and recognition of interpersonal concerns and attunement to those concerns become visible only when things go wrong. For example, a student gave an account of being in a situation where her skills of involvement were not yet sufficient for the patient's needs:

I remember the second quarter, we took Effective Communication, and we talked about communication and about what you should do in different situations. I found myself in a situation in a room where a woman was very upset because she had cancer ... she just had surgery and she was worried how her husband would feel about the disfigurement to her body. She thought he was really upset. It was such a surreal experience because I found myself sitting in there thinking, "All right, now I'm supposed to be an active listener and supposed to reflect the questions." So I felt like I was doing it by textbook. And I'm thinking, "This is someone's life, and I'm sitting here and I'm doing this and no one's watching me." I felt really over my head ... but that's what we do. We're in people's lives and our job and our role is affecting people's lives. I still remember that experience, and now in my practice it comes a lot more naturally, but I remember that very clearly; I remember thinking, "What do I do? What action do I take?"

I remember the side of the bed I was sitting on. She was just really sad and really depressed, and she was just crying. We learned you're supposed to say, "Are you feeling sad?" And it came out of my mouth. I thought, "Oh, it seems like the right thing to say, because that's what I'm supposed to do." And I said that thing, but it was kind of awkward ... but I was the only one there; I was the only one talking to her. So I think it did help to some extent, but I still felt very awkward doing it, and she was definitely more caught up in her emotions and really sad and was crying and she probably didn't notice my ineptitude.... She responded. She said, "Yes, I am feeling sad," and she kind of elaborated. I don't know if I was anticipating her emotions, but I sensed that she started to sense that I didn't know what I was doing. [laughs] And she started to withdraw.... I remember feeling like she was starting to close up, not open up, but she had this big open-up and then stopped. She kind of sensed that I was in over my head.

Students must learn to distinguish when communication techniques are useful and when presence and compassion are the most one can offer. The student recalls the feeling of being "in over my head" and sensing a patient withdraw because she was not comfortable in the situation. This is a moment of insight and experiential learning that has an impact on the student as she reflects on it.

Students learn what kinds of emotional involvement they can engage in concerning their patient's problems and the kinds of emotional connection that work well for the patient and nurse. At its most elementary, this is called *boundary work*, in which the student learns where to stand emotionally with the patient. In learning boundaries with patients, students learn not to merge with the patient's plight or pain or overidentify with the patient. They must also learn not to be too objective, too distant, but to be sufficiently open to the patient's experience to understand the patient's concerns and be of help. In addition to learning these skills of involvement, students must learn to refine their skills with patients, how they approach and care for patients, how they help their patients manage their illness, or how they help patients express concerns about their illness or health. Appropriate skills of involvement for the patient situation and patient concerns have to be learned experientially through reflecting on when the relationship went well and when it did not go so well, much as the student who knew that she was in over her head did. As one educator stated, "The issue around communicating with patients who have emotional pain is so essential." Many students must learn to be with patients who experience a depth of suffering that before they started nursing school they could not have imagined:

> A very crucial moment for me occurred when I was doing my medical-surgical rotation. It was our fall quarter and I was in a room with a family where the husband had been newly diagnosed, he was young, with end-stage colon cancer. He had been admitted for pain control. The primary oncologist called on the phone, which was probably not a very good way for the wife to get this news. He told the wife that whatever treatment option they thought they might be able to do wasn't going to be an option anymore and they had to start thinking about hospice. I just happened to be in the room when she was talking on the phone with him and sort of just experienced . . . I mean, I was totally caught off guard and not prepared to deal with something like that.
>
> She hung up the phone and it was obvious that she was upset, so I think I must have asked her what had happened, and she immediately just opened up, started crying and the husband was pretty unresponsive from the amount of pain medication they had given him and was a little confused, so the patient wasn't very active in the conversation. It was just me mostly hugging her while she was crying and just trying to help her through that as much as I could, while clearly being in over my head and not knowing what I was doing.

"Caught off guard," the student learned by accident an important lesson about the intimate demands of being present with someone during moments of crisis and grief and just being present, not offering advice, not fleeing.

Strategies for Teaching Skills of Perception and Involvement

Students learn skills of involvement most powerfully when engaged with patients, families, and other professionals in specific clinical situations where they can develop attuned perceptions and astute clinical assessments. They can also learn relational skills of involvement in simulation and direct patient care. We found that skills of involvement and discussions of caring practices were noticeably absent in the classrooms that we observed. Two effective pedagogies of clinical teaching, reflection and coaching, are promising strategies for bringing these experiences into the classroom as well.

Many nurse educators draw on the concept of reflective practice (Schön, 1987) by asking their students to write reflective journals (Lasater & Nielson, 2009). Students reflect on the perceptions and emotions that come up for them during clinical experiences, and the teacher coaches the students in developing effective skills of involvement with patients:

> Many of us have picked up on having students write journals. I'll say to them, "I don't want to know about how many ideas you had or what you did. I want to know about what that experience meant to you. Tell me." And I write back to them and engage in a dialogue because in the acute pediatric care setting, you're not going to have time for that. For example, one student wrote about not feeling much compassion for a baby on a ventilator. The student wrote, "I'm thinking that this little baby eventually was going to get off the vent and unlike that older adult who probably was going to die on the vent. Am I heartless because I didn't have all these feelings of compassion in my heart for the infant on the vent? What's wrong with me?" ... I wrote back and said, "You know one person's threat is another's challenge. The ventilator was a temporary challenge for the infant.... Because you didn't have this overwhelming emotional response to this little premature baby on a vent doesn't make you a heartless individual. It's just that you're going to come across experiences that you approach differently on an emotional level." And we talked about that. I would have [had] no idea that this was her experience or if she felt that way had it not been for the reflective journal.

Initially the student imagines that she should have the same level and kind of emotional response to what looked like similar situations to her. The teacher helped her articulate her own intuitions about being temporarily on a ventilator at the beginning of life and the suffering involved as a result of permanently being on a ventilator at the end of life. The student needs to understand that her seeming "lack of compassion" for the infant does not make her "heartless," or even indicate that she is truly lacking compassion, but rather represents a hopeful and engaged connection with the infant's future possibilities. This process of clarification and articulation can help the students better understand their emotional responses and skills of engagement. A teacher recalls a student who was in a psychiatric setting: "The patient told her he was HIV positive. She described in her journal not wanting to touch him, and she was afraid. She said: "'I feel very bad that I felt that way'. . . I was glad that she expressed her feelings so she could work through them. In psychiatric nursing, we have guidelines for them to describe the experience. I pretty much try to make the students stick to that so they do not just use it in a cursory sort of way."

Without the formal space given to reflecting on interpersonal engagement and emotional responses, the student would have perhaps kept private what were to her shameful feelings of fear and avoidance. Through sharing and confronting feelings, students have a greater chance of working through their prejudices in dialogue with a supportive teacher.

Coaching

Clinical faculty guide students in learning to develop their skills of perception and involvement by questioning them about issues of salience: asking what the students are paying attention to and how they understand what they are seeing in the clinical setting. As one educator explained, "When I evaluate the students' performance, I'm looking for them to be paying attention to the right things. And the only way I can know that is if they tell me what they're paying attention to. Sometimes the problem is not so much that they aren't paying attention to the right things, but just that they can't articulate what they are paying attention to. So, I coach them through that, to help them figure it out: 'Well, wait now. I'm not understanding you. It seems like you're on the wrong track here.'"

The nurse educator, focusing on the students' sense of salience, coaches them to make explicit the subtle cues that they may never have seen or understood before in a clinical situation. For this faculty member, what the student is noticing is as much a question or source of curiosity as an observation of the student's performance of a technical skill. Helping the student articulate these tentative observations is the only way to discover the student's sense of the situation. For the student, gaining good descriptive language about what he is seeing in the patient's condition or situation is crucial to the process of forming and articulating good clinical judgments.

Taking Responsibility

Many students described a pivotal learning situation, a moment when they experienced the deep responsibilities of being a nurse. We noted that an important feature of their narratives about these crucial experiences was the realization of not only their deep responsibilities but also their ability to act effectively in these situations. The students' ability to integrate knowledge, skilled know-how, and ethical comportment contributed to an important transformation in their self-understanding and identity.

Some students grasped the significance of their responsibility through a situation where the accident of their presence made the difference:

> My first real eye-opening experience was on medical-surgical rotation, junior year. We were on a general medical unit, and I don't remember what was wrong with the patient because I never got a chance to get report. I came to clinical that day and I was feeling really sick. I was very nauseated and spent the first fifteen minutes in the bathroom. When I came out and told my professor, she said, "OK, you have two patients today, and one is going down for a test, so you don't even have to do anything with her. For your other patient, just go wait for report and see how you're feeling. If you want to lie down, you may." I was waiting for report and I glanced in the room and I could hear her, she was having agonal breathing. So I walked in the room and she was breathing but she was not responsive. The physician walked in at that point and he stood there for five minutes trying to wake her up, and she wasn't waking. So I went and got the pulse oximeter and her oxygen percentage was 60. So we called the code and they gave her Narcan and she came back. And then they transferred her to the ICU. That really hit me because I hadn't even received the report yet. I knew nothing about his patient; I didn't even know her name. And within five minutes we were already so close to the possibility of someone dying.... And it blew me away—the power that nurses have when they're with patients, to really save them.... She was a postoperative surgery patient. I know that she had had too much morphine. She had a PCA [patient-controlled analgesia] and I guess they had given her a bolus that was too much for her.

The experience drew the student's attention to the capability that she has, being able to integrate knowledge and skilled action in the interest of doing what is best for the patient. The student realized that the patient was in danger and acted immediately on her discovery; her quick recognition and action in assessing the patient's oxygen level clarified the diagnosis of opiate overdose. Her skill of assessing oxygen saturation, where to find the necessary equipment, how to use it, and how to interpret the results were integrated with her immediate recognition of the patient's breathing as dangerously abnormal. Because she acted "as a nurse would act," she made a difference to the patient, who could easily have been overlooked during the busy "end of shift report" time. This student grew in her belief that as a nurse she must be vigilant and respond quickly and responsibly to patient distress.

Other students learned the import of their actions by glimpsing the tragic consequences of another choice:

> I had this experience on our first day in the Mother, Baby, Labor, and Delivery course. My professor said, "OK, Jennifer, you're going to have two couplets today. You're going to have four patients," and, back then, that was a big deal. So I was running around, head down. I did the assessments, and I was really getting nervous because it was getting late and I still hadn't assessed the last baby yet. I walked into the nursery and the nurse there said, "Oh, don't worry about that baby. I just assessed her and everything's fine." And I remember standing there thinking, "Oh, good." But then I said, "I can't do that," you know, I can't do that. *You can't do that*.... I opened up the blanket and looked in and sure enough, the baby was tachycardic, flaccid, and cold. That's the day I realized the awesome responsibility to do our job because that baby was then placed in the incubator and Intensive Care and was there for at least a week. And I'm thinking, "How many hours would it have been 'til somebody had actually discovered the baby's condition?" Had I just listened to the staff nurse, as a student, and said "OK, the RN said she assessed the baby now, and she had documented her assessment"—but just because it was my patient assignment, as a student, I still had to go and do it [the assessment]. It was a good feeling to realize, hey, I really can actually assess an infant and find something wrong. And I think that's the day I realized that you are responsible. I don't care if somebody else has that assignment. If you have anything to do with that patient, you're responsible.... It was a day I realized that *even that early on* you're very important... I still remember that day. So, every day I go in to do assessment, I think, "Nope, I'm doing everything. I don't care, head to toe. We're not skipping over anything." That was an important day.... They give you the tools and you really just have to go in there and do it, and even though there are time constraints, and there are always time constraints as a

student, it's worth getting in trouble for being behind rather than to
put your patients' care in jeopardy. That was an important lesson.

The stakes were high; the infant's life was truly in the student's hands.
The staff nurse may have been correct in her earlier assessment of the
infant; infants can change rapidly. The import of the event is that the student learned, firsthand, that she must take responsibility for her patients.
No nursing educator intentionally plans such a risky learning experience. Even so, similar situations will likely repeat in other settings and
with other patients in most students' clinical experience. This experience
formed part of this student's habitus, her way of being a nurse and a person in the world, and a new set of perceptual capacities associated with
ways to respond both to the routines a nurse is expected to enact (always
assessing your own patients) and respond quickly to unexpected clinical
concerns (finding the baby flaccid and cold).

In the course of her narrative, the student illustrates how she drew on all
three dimensions of learning. The ethical comportment she is developing
is evident: she reminded herself of her responsibility to do what she was
responsible for. She noted the baby was tachycardic, knowledge gained
from physiology, and flaccid, a clinical judgment learned in the physical
assessment skills laboratory. She also grasped immediately that it was
imperative to act quickly and efficiently, with her focus on doing all that
she could for the baby. The experience further reinforced her sense of
responsibility: "So, every day I go in to do assessment, I think, 'Nope,
I'm doing everything. I don't care, head to toe. We're not skipping over
anything.'"

We highlight these powerful, identity-conferring experiences that students shared as central to their formation because we see that these
practices need attention in the classroom and should not be left to the
chance of clinical experience alone. These formative experiences are too
important to be left to chance. We were distressed to find that nurse educators generally confine the opportunity for such experiences to the clinical
situation. In general, the nursing curriculum is constructed so that knowledge and technical skills are presented in ways that do not ask the students
to imagine using that knowledge in concrete clinical situations. Such a separation of knowledge acquisition and use encourages nursing educators
to overlook the need to integrate the dimensions of learning for practice and to use teaching strategies that do not require students to use
the knowledge they are learning. Indeed, it was not surprising to us that
teachers often recounted stories about students who performed well in
the classroom and on tests of formal knowledge but failed in the clinical

setting because they could not use the formal knowledge in underdetermined, ambiguous, and constantly changing clinical situations involving relationships with patients, their families, and other clinicians.

We recommend more articulation and appreciation in the classroom of nursing's central focal practices, such as attentiveness and vigilance, so that students have meaningful opportunities to develop clinical and moral imagination by rehearsing, in a safe setting, how they integrate their knowledge, skilled know-how, and ethical comportment, and contemplating the obligations of being a nurse. As Diane Pestolesi, Lisa Day, Sarah Shannon, and other teachers we observed demonstrate, in the classroom students can learn ethical comportment for excellent care of their patients. To prepare students for the complex, underdetermined, and ill-defined clinical situations where nurses practice, teachers must create opportunities for active learning, where students confront gaps in their knowledge and previously unexamined assumptions. In such classes they can forge connections and develop clinical imagination. Shannon, for example, uses dialogical and consciousness-raising strategies in her ethics class that encourage self-disclosure and discovery. She creates a safe space and safe ways for students to confront their assumptions and biases.

Focal Practices of Nursing

Formation is *caught* as well taught. Japanese educators would call this learning by osmosis (Sagara, 2003). We now know that learning usually occurs in the context of membership and participation in a community of learning or practice. Communities and human beings need care, and acting on that need is a focal practice of nursing. Focal practices reinforce what is central to a particular subset of meanings, practices, and telos of a socially embedded practice (Borgmann, 1984). Cultures have focal practices such as weddings and funerals, and families have focal practices that gather them together such as family meals, shared sports, and so on. Focal practices both gather up existing meanings and extend those meanings in specific instances in a practice such as nursing, or social meanings and practices within a professional practice, a culture, or family.

The story of the compassionate stranger in the Christian New Testament (Wuthnow, 1993) and similar stories in other cultures convey common notions that persons are member-participants of a common humanity. Buddhism has strong notions of compassion and caring for others instantiated by Buddha. Common to all human beings is that they are finite, embodied, and interdependent and therefore require support and care throughout the life cycle; these and many others are existing cultural meanings and moral sources that nurses extend into their practice. Judaism has a strong tradition of *Tikkun Olam*, which refers to repairing the world or engaging in social justice, which is often lodged in healing practices of health care or *gemilut hasadim* (acts of kindness; My Jewish Learning, n.d.). Cultural traditions have their own focal practices that gather up the meanings of care and social responsibility. Nursing as a social practice and tradition has focal practices that embody the meanings of caring for the other in health, vulnerability, or illness.

Learning nursing's focal practices, such as being present for patients and bearing witness to their suffering, patient advocacy, and responsibility, are central to formation of the nurse, and they are also formative of practice and learning communities in nursing. Focal practices in nursing contain a cluster of caring practices that nurses consider central to their understanding of nursing and their identity as nurses. For example, patient advocacy includes giving the silent patient a voice, ensuring medical treatments are manageable and do not conflict with patient concerns and intentions. Being present for a patient may entail holding a child, or sitting with a patient until the pain medication takes hold, or staying by the patient's head soothing and talking the person through a difficult procedure or passage. Bearing witness to patient and family suffering, recovery, or illness experience is a form of being present that includes such actions as keeping track of improvement; recognizing, assessing, and negotiating comfort measures and pain management; or assisting the patient in maintaining spiritual practices during a hospitalization (Benner, 2000; Benner et al., 1999).

Nursing students gave us many accounts of experiential learning that transformed their sense of identity. Eight themes that emerged from senior nursing students' stories of significant experiential learning are summarized here:

1. *Formation stories were often a major singular theme in the senior's narratives.* However, themes of formation were also woven into many of the stories, as students acknowledged how a particular learning experience had changed their perspective, their capacity to act in a similar situation in the future, their self-knowledge, and their understanding, or had reassured them that they were on the right path and that they were going to be good at their chosen profession.

2. *Meeting and treating the patient as a person* rather than as a patient, or object of care. These stories of learning were the most frequent themes for nursing students who were preoccupied in the beginning

of their practice with technical intervention, patient safety, and knowledge and skills of patient assessment and response to therapy. In their stories, it was as if the patient as a person suddenly claimed their attention and reframed their ethical comportment. They responded with a mixture of discovery and chagrin over their having been overly focused on the technical.

3. Recognizing the patient first as a person led the student to efforts to *preserve the patient's personhood and dignity in the face of the ravages of injuries, illness, and the influence of many medications.* The students learned to highlight the person's social and family identity as a recognition practice for the family and for the staff. They often used pictures from the patient's life, humor, and stories of outside everyday life to help capture the person's social identity.

4. *The fear of making a mistake*, the recognition of the level of responsibility of nursing practice, that a nurse's actions could seriously harm or even cause death were major formative themes of nursing students. The students' lay expectations of a nurse as helper had not included the high precision and knowledge-skill actually required by nurses. Student nurses told stories of making mistakes, of reporting their errors, and of their terror at the possibility of making a more dangerous mistake.

5. *Learning technical skills* was a major theme in most of the narratives; however, many of the student's stories took the form of telling their anticipatory fear of inserting an IV, of assisting with hemodialysis, inserting a nasogastric tube, and their relief over successfully accomplishing the technical feat and then having it recede in the background with more experience.

6. Stories of *effective staff nurse or teacher coaching in difficult clinical situations* that enabled the student to take responsibility and experience independence while performing a difficult clinical intervention were also told as stories of formation through taking on the identity of a nurse in an actual clinical setting. Students were relieved when their teachers protected their sense of professional identity in front of the patient. They also appreciated teachers' preparatory coaching outside the room as well, because it gave them the opportunity to take up and feel responsible for the patient.

7. *Confronting substandard care in hospital settings* and the ethical challenges to report substandard care were major themes for the student nurses who hold a low-status position in a rigid hospital

hierarchy. Students usually went to their nurse educators for support and correction and were then met with a range of satisfactory corrective responses, or less satisfactory advice "not to make waves" because students are precarious guests in the hospital, and clinical placements are hard to find.

8. *Difficulties in making the transition to work* loomed large for all the senior students. When one student told of her concerns about the first job, other students chimed in and agreed, adding their own fears. Many stories focused on fear of not being prepared to move competently into the work role. Seniors wanted to find good institutional cultures and hoped to find residencies or specialized training for newly graduated nurses.

These major themes of senior nursing students' narratives of experiential learning capture focal practices in nursing and impediments to fully realizing these focal practices.

Meeting the Patient as a Person

To be with a patient and bear witness to the patient's plight is one of the focal caring practices of nurses. A student describes bearing witness to a patient's suffering and providing alternative comfort measures for a patient who was writhing in pain but could not have more pain medication at that moment: "The nurse that had this patient didn't have time to be with her at that time, and I thought: 'I've got to do something,' and we couldn't give her anything else [for pain]. We had just given her pain medication, and we're waiting for it to take effect. I thought: 'I have to be with this person and witness her pain, and I held her hand. I had the other nurse turn down the lights, and I just talked to her and helped her do guided imagery to get through that difficult time." The student nurse knew that she needed to be present for the patient and not abandon her during this difficult time.

We were impressed with the evidence of the focal practices of nursing in the narratives of senior students who told about their pivotal learning experiences in their clinical practice. Being present, preserving the personhood of acutely ill or injured persons, and many other accounts of meeting a patient as a person reveal the extent to which these focal practices contribute to student formation. It is remarkable and laudable that these focal practices survive in the current context of market-driven health care systems, although they are dangerously marginalized in many settings. Unfortunately, attention to these central, identity-conferring practices were all but absent in formal classroom lectures. However, they are firmly present in clinical education; focal practices were evident primarily in student narratives of meaningful nursing experiences, in students' clinical journals, and in the clinical debriefing sessions we observed in all nine nursing programs that we visited.

Preserving Personhood

Preserving personhood in a highly bureaucratic environment where patients and family members feel vulnerable is another facet of meeting the patient as a person, and patient advocacy. A student explained:

> For some reason there's always one patient who gets left out because there are too many patients for a nurse to deal with. It didn't help the fact that this patient specifically had a little mild dementia. When the nurse would walk in there, she would say things to her and the patient would go, "Ay, ay, ay." Just in and out and that was it. And I just felt like, "That's not patient care!" So I took it upon myself to go in there and talk to her and just do her daily cares. Every now and then she'd ask, "Where am I? Can I go outside?" She just wanted to be around people and just wanted to talk to somebody. And by the end of the day, her husband came in and she told him how good she felt that day. And that just made a difference. She really reminds you also that these people are real people and that you need to be treating them as human beings.

Another student remarked on learning about care for the elderly and praised her gerontology class for instilling in her the importance of providing care that preserves the dignity and worth of the elderly: "I think something else that was valuable was our gerontology class and learning to deal with geriatric patients and realizing they're people, too. Because so many times they're not treated the way they should be treated and they're not given respect . . . in that class, especially the film that we had to watch . . . you sit there and you're in tears, and the way this lady was treated. It makes you realize you don't want to be that way. I think that was important, too, in the beginning."

Patient Advocacy

The focal practice most frequently articulated by students and teachers is patient advocacy. We present it after "meeting the patient as a person" and preserving personhood, only because it cannot logically happen in any attuned way unless the patient is met and understood by the nurse. The tradition of patient advocacy is nested in a long and textured set of relational and caring practices, and it includes the notion of legal and ethical responsibility for the patient and family, who may not be able to advocate for themselves for lack of knowledge or incapacitation through illness or grief. As one educator explained, "We all teach the psychosocial aspects of nursing, and professionalism, and advocacy for patients. And sometimes the advocacy is not asking the physician for an order, or advocating for this type of diet for the patient. Sometimes it's helping the patients speak for themselves. And either being there, supporting the patients, or reminding the patients of questions they wanted to bring to the physician."

In the eyes of students and teachers alike, patient advocacy is linked with care and comfort as well as with empowerment, as this educator explained:

> A student has to be a patient advocate, and this has to begin with the very beginning. It has to begin in the first semester. She has to understand that her role is very noble, to be there at the patient bedside, and she has to recognize that safe practice might not be provided by some. She has to speak for the patient what is unspeakable, for the patient who is in a coma, for the intubated patient. The whole role is to prevent the patient from any injury and disability. She has to be the guardian of patient care. We try to instill that into them right from the beginning. It is again a very long process. It doesn't happen in the first semester. You introduce, you begin, and you build on it, and you monitor the student, and you help her to understand why she is there in the first place. You know that she has many hats that she's wearing and has many roles that she has to fulfill.

Although patient advocacy is fragile because it must be enacted amid multiple demands, it is perhaps the glue that holds hospital care together, making it safer than it would be without the nurse's commitment to vigilance and advocacy (Thomas, 1995). It is worth noting the ubiquity of the notion of patient advocacy in nursing education: it is the very fabric of nursing education and practice. One educator commented how it is fully incorporated into the curriculum, even to assessment: "We look at whether or not they support the clients in their decisions and then advocate for their rights and entitlement to quality nursing practice. We focus on advocacy in this particular course. Each course has something on the human caring relationship, which is where our advocacy piece comes from."

A student described how she has learned to empathize and extend her understanding of the patient's and family's plight at the end of life: "One of the ways that the school has nurtured empathy is in the emphasis on pain of patients, always letting us know: 'Turning the patient causes the most pain among patients in the hospital.' Also, palliative care and emphasizing the comfort of the patient and also telling us about families and loved ones, how what affects them most is how their loved one died. Were they in pain, or were they comfortable? And I've seen that as a common theme of all our classes."

Pedagogies for Patient Advocacy

Teaching about patient advocacy begins with meeting the patient, recognizing the person at the end of the bed—and it must begin early. As a step toward meeting the patient, for example, we observed a number of skills labs where teachers ask students to understand the patient's experience of receiving treatments and toileting. As one student commented, "The other really good thing about lab is that in skills lab the faculty make you *feel* like the patient. So, when you're in the hospital and you're putting a bed pan under your butt, lying in bed you know first-hand what it is like. Now we know what that feels like and how bed baths feel, too."

To help students put patients into the context of the world in which they live, some teachers bring former patients and family members into the classroom so that students can understand the human issues related to coping with an illness, disability, or rehabilitation:

EDUCATOR 1: I bring in a patient, and I have the patient focus on one of the three lectures. It's sort of pulling all three lectures of the whole gamut of cardiovascular disease. I ask the patient what made a difference in their stay.... The patient was tearful last year. I've known him for three or four years. I never thought this man would cry in front of a group of 130 nursing students. He got tearful when he explained what made a difference with nursing. And so even in that small way if we can bring the patient's experience into the classroom it helps the students to understand.

EDUCATOR 2: We do the same kind of thing in our course. Last week we were focusing on chronic illness and developmental disabilities and hemophilia as disease. And a mother of a child with Down syndrome, who also is a pediatric nurse, was invited to teach for a short period of time about Down syndrome and about having a child with Down syndrome. Speaking of tears, at the end of the class she read the story about a trip to

Europe. There were so many difficulties in a relatively ordinary trip. Well by the time she finished that the students were all crying, she was crying, I was crying.

EDUCATOR 3: The word *advocate* has been used by several people here, and that's just crucial and it's key that you are responsible for this person, that you are their voice. And so, that's absolutely been stressed by this program, and I think by nursing in general.

There seems to be a tacit agreement between students and clinical teachers that effective patient advocacy requires understanding patients' context, their world, and their experience. Clinical educators encouraged students to sit down and get to know the patient as a person, and understand the meanings of the illness for the patient and the family. They asked students to talk about their patients in the postclinical conferences, engaging them so that they would arrive at a deeper understanding of the patient's experiences. However, with a few exceptions, including beyond those cited here, the classroom unfortunately was not a site for this type of contextualized pedagogy around patient advocacy or focal nursing practices. If students did speak about the experiences of their patients in the classroom, it was briefly and either in answer to a directed question from the teacher or as a question for the teacher.

Pedagogies of contextualization help the student appreciate the patients' illnesses in the context of their lives. Such strategies stand in stark contrast to the pedagogies of objectification and decontextualization that are often deployed in teaching the natural science of physiology and disease, doing assessments, performing painful procedures, or assisting in surgery. This decontextualization and objectification is the language of biomedicine, where both nurse and physician clinicians seek to isolate the "disease" or "pathophysiology" at the cellular or system level apart from the patient's everyday experiences. For example, when poverty, smoking, or alcohol consumption are included in a history and physical, these aspects of patient and family life are stripped of their context and discussed as isolated "risk factors" that can be reduced through medical or social intervention. Yet regardless of the risk factor modification strategies used, patients continue to dwell in their world with their concerns and projects. Nurses are instructed to do "holistic" patient assessments where the patient's significant others, family, and life context show up. Specific strategies to elicit this kind of information are absolutely essential to nurses who understand themselves as patient advocates in hospital, clinic, and community practice settings.

Attention to patient experience yields patient advocacy such as that described by a student who spoke about learning the difference that a nurse can make when she meets "as a person" someone seriously ill or near death:

> This man's care was very difficult and hard to manage. He had tubes. He had liver cancer, so he had J tubes. He had tubes everywhere and he was older. His family was there, and so when I walked in, I introduced myself. It was like he had the wall up already. And so I thought, "Well, I'm going to try a different strategy." So I pulled up a chair and sat next to him, and I introduced myself. He had pictures from his grandkids and I have kids, so I just kind of started the conversation and he was saying that he really misses them and they couldn't come and see him because of the procedure. And then I was talking about the weather. I just kind of wanted to break the hospital surroundings and what he was missing. And I said, "You know, this is all new to me. I have a lot of stuff to do. You're my primary care person"…and he said, "Thank you very much for talking. You know, you're the first person that's treated me as a person." So it was like I put him on a level of a person and then when I was fumbling, doing first-semester fumbling with all kinds of stuff—fumbling with the gowns, fumbling with PO meds, checking all the bands, making sure he was all safe and doing all that kind of stuff—he just was a person.
>
> And so when I went back the next week, I got an order so that he could take a shower with his tubes. We wrapped the tubes and we locked [the] bathroom door … it was an hour-long process for him to take a shower. And the next week I went in and he was dying. And his family came up and said, "You know what? Out of all the people that have been here, you were the one that he trusted because you kept it on a personal level. You sat down next to him, not on his bed, and he was more of a person."
>
> So ever since then I've always made it a habit of at least talking a little bit to the patients so that they're just not a number and you do care. The empathy is there and it's made a difference. And so it was hard because that was the first patient I took care of that died, but it taught me a lot.

This experience of meeting the patient as a person bears a family resemblance to many such student nurse encounters. As the student becomes attentive in the moment or present for the patient, such experiences can occur more frequently. The student will seek them out, learning to listen in order to meet the patient and informally acknowledge the patient's personhood and plight. This recognition practice is at the heart of nursing's focal practices. Students' narratives indicate that they often come to these high-level interpersonal skills rather late in their program. Students want to continue to improve their ability to meet the patient as a person and bear witness to the patient's illness experience, only to discover that they have to fight to preserve their time. They develop these caring practices, despite being pushed for efficiency and being daunted by heavy workloads.

We now turn, in the next chapter, to those ever-present institutional pressures that marginalize caring practices and in turn exert their own formative press on the student's identity, skills, and character.

12

FORMATION FROM A CRITICAL STANCE

WE NOTED THAT patient advocacy was often taught explicitly in the context of encountering substandard nursing practice. The powerful and sometimes dysfunctional roles of our health care institutions can have undesirable consequences for the formation and practice of nurses. At the policy level, health care institutions need to be made more hospitable and fit for good nursing and medical practice. But, if used as a teaching-learning opportunity, substandard practice can be used to inoculate students with the frontline issues in nursing, and be a source for thinking realistically about change strategies to improve practice.

Nursing students learn in complex, bureaucratic settings with economic constraints and limited resources, where the goals of the institution may clash with the goals of good professional practice. As one student explained:

> I learned how hard nursing is. I saw a lot of tired nurses, too, on my floor. I think that's good to see, too, to just be aware of, to keep myself healthy, to keep myself happy. The nurses are amazing, but they are worked, and a lot are tired. There aren't any real breaks for a nurse. Someone can take a fifteen-minute break and walk down and get a cup of coffee, but a nurse has to stay on that floor. I can't tell you how many cups of coffee I saw with only three sips out of them because a patient in room seven was vomiting, or something else happens, like a patient's IV came out in room ten. It was an eye-opener.

In fact, none of the senior students we interviewed were leaving school without having had their "eyes opened" to the demands of the acute-care hospital and long-term care environments. It is clear from our interviews that improving working environments is central to any solution to the nursing shortage and to improving patient care and safety. Equally essential is addressing the substandard practice and dysfunctional work environments for students' potential learning about change, and preparing themselves to cope with the realities of what they are likely to confront at work when they graduate. Exposure to substandard work environments can also help students identify health care delivery systems that present a better work environment.

In any health care practice, the professional must make efforts to influence the institutional context so that good practice is feasible within the bureaucratic and economic limits and organizational infrastructures of the practice setting. As one teacher pointed out, the challenge of facing patients with critical illness is compounded by the demands of the large complex bureaucratic settings in which care takes place:

> I think they struggle in the clinical the most ... just see what they see in the clinical setting. For a lot of them, it's the first time they've seen people as sick as these people are, and the first time they've seen people dying or families in distress, and it's really hard. And it's the first time for some of them to see the big institution of acute care. That acute tertiary care setting is really challenging for a lot of the students, just to be in there. The communication that goes on there and the expectations and how patients are treated and how families are treated ... just seeing this whole structure and how many problems there are with it. So, the discussions that we have in clinical conferences include what's wrong with the system and what's wrong with acute care and why people are so sick in the hospital. That seems to be the part that they find most challenging.... But for some of them it's the first time they've been in the environment for an extended period. And then, they have to function there. So it's not just that they're there observing and looking and saying, "My god, look at this place. It's really scary and dysfunctional and has a lot of problems." They have to navigate these problems and get through that and do the best they can for their patients.

In the face of such health care inequities, students must learn how to better understand the patient's context and how they can help patients improve their access and continuity of care. Advocating for the under-served and uninsured is a major focus of patient advocacy in the student and interviews with educators. For example, advocacy for patients on discharge is a major theme in student comments. Frequently students told stories of giving elaborate discharge teaching and instructions, only to find out that the patient was unable to afford the medications, was without insurance, or was homeless. There was no easy solution for follow-up care after extensive surgery. Commenting on such experiences, one student observed, "Our health care system isn't perfect, and we want to try to be advocates for our patients, and I think learning about these things helps me figure out how I can exert my influence on behalf of my patients." Another noted: "I work at a trauma center. It's also a place that serves disadvantaged people, both jail patients, illegal immigrants, people that have newly migrated, and just having an appreciation for the system they've come from, their frame of mind, the system that they're in, what benefits they're going to get, and having some insight into their situation and maybe what's in store for them helps me to advocate for them in their situation."

In the best situation, the institution facilitates good practice as defined by the professionals working in the institution. The boundaries of good and poor practice are set not only by the performance, skill, and integrity of the professionals but also by the organizational context that supports or constrains best practices. The importance of patient advocacy showed up vividly when student nurses confronted substandard nursing care: patient neglect, or labeling patients as difficult, or even verbal abuse. In these areas of the breakdown or breach of good practice, the students could identify loss of patient advocacy and feel its significance for patient well-being powerfully. Teachers tried to help them:

> We see practice that is less than wonderful. We see nurses who treat patients badly and nurses who don't tell the truth to patients and things like that. And we talk a lot about, How do you deal with that when you're a nurse? What do you do with that and how do you, as an RN on the treatment team, help LVNs [licensed vocational nurses], aides, and other RNs to look at their practice and maybe be able to make some changes? How do you do that in a way that you can be heard? How do you do that if you don't have any institutional authority because you don't have institutional authority the first few years you're in practice? How do you use yourself to help to make changes in the professionalism of people?

Nurse educators must prepare students to face intransigent bureaucracies bent on cutting costs, and with little or no appreciation of the nurse's role in making patient care safe and technologies bearable. Efforts include leadership courses, often part of BSN programs, which typically emphasize issues of practice and policy reform, especially related to patient safety (Cronenwett et al., 2007). Students are often assigned "change projects" such as introducing the latest evidence-based care for IV changes and site

care, translation of patient education booklets into Spanish, identifying
resources for homeless people such as mobile clinics, lobbying to ensure
that mouth shields are in every room for mouth-to-mouth resuscitation,
or calling an ethical consultation meeting about a common violation of
patients' right to informed consent. We noted that nurse educators understood both formal and informal change projects as addressing the nurse's
role as change agent for patient's well-being.

   We found educators and students who resist many forces for dehu-
manization in hospitalization. We heard impressive examples of students
advocating for patients in circumstances of practice breakdown. One student who witnessed the verbal abuse of a patient by a nurse who had
worked a number of shifts in a row intervened with the patient, and then
again at the system level—successfully, because she was supported by her
clinical instructor and preceptor. An RN taking her BSN described the
problems she had with a nursing manager who did not act on requests
for more staff in a pediatric day surgery recovery room:

> We told the nurse manager over and over we needed more help to be
> safe but we were told to get to the phone and call for help when needed.
> It didn't work. She wouldn't understand that. We had an incident
> where it got really out of control. We called for help. We ended up with
> more people in there than we needed. Fortunately, nobody got hurt
> except for the mother.... This one ear, nose, and throat [ENT] doctor
> works out of two rooms, so you have two different anesthesia persons
> giving these kids anesthesia gases and they wake up at different stages.
> In addition, a bone marrow transplant surgeon's time is eight minutes
> so those children could hit the recovery room in fifteen minutes. Then,
> you have your next ENT coming out in another fifteen minutes, so the
> kid doesn't have time to emerge from anesthesia. One minute they're
> sleeping and the next minute they're jumping over the rail of the crib.
> Never mind, if it's not a life-threatening airway problem or an adverse
> drug reaction, etc.
>
>   We don't have a phone within our reach, so we have to leave the
> recovery room and go to the phone. You have one person to keep the
> person's baby safe and they split the parents up, so you have to find
> the parents, and then you have the one come in and then you've got to
> play all your different roles. You've got to explain to the mother that
> the child's safe. Never mind not even keeping IV sites intact and the
> kid's screaming and you have to give medications.
>
>   So, the next child came in, we had two nurses. The other child was
> settled in the mother's arms. The other child came out and he was

ballistic. All the issues that the parents deal with at home like behavioral problems come out when the child is coming out of anesthesia. The child wasn't in a state where he could be reasoned with. We didn't have any help. The mother came in by accident because a volunteer brought her in. So, we put the mother on a stretcher, she's holding her child, well he's still not in a state where he could be reasoned with. . . . Anesthesia had brought him out and said give him Demerol. So, we're giving Demerol IV and I had given him 20 mg of Demerol already in 5 mg increments. We had two children in there, two mothers, and two nurses. I put the mother on the stretcher with the child in her arms, still not settling after 20 mg of Demerol. The child bit the mother so hard that he was latched on and we could not separate. So, finally we get the help we need and it's a big fiasco. The mother's out crying. I said to somebody: "Don't leave that mother alone. We will deal with the child." Finally I get a nurse to hold that child and by then the Demerol had been absorbed from the infiltrated IV site. And then the child settled, but it was just so needless, all caused by lack of adequate staffing.

In response to this incident, the nurse wrote a powerful letter, describing the incident, with a clear analysis of the problem of staffing. She then clearly outlined her requests for correcting the problem. In response to this persuasive and clear analysis of this dangerous staffing problem, the chief of anesthesia responded: "You have my support in anything you ask for." He said, "That letter was appropriate. It was not accusing." He had heard my verbal request before, but this time he really understood the problem.

The student said that it would not have occurred to her to write the letter and enlist the support of her colleagues before a leadership course in her BSN completion program. She had newfound confidence in her writing skills and understood her actions as effective advocacy for the children's safety. One hallmark of ethical comportment in any professional practice is commitment to influence institutional policies that govern professional knowledge-based practice. Nursing students need to be better prepared to speak in health care and organizational policy arenas.

Nursing's Social Contract: Civic Professionalism

The high expectations for "acting like a nurse" that we saw stressed in nursing programs is a form of civic professionalism (Sullivan, 2005), a vision that can be linked back to Aristotle's observation that a practice such as being a statesman is different from what can be accomplished solely by rules and procedures. A practice requires knowledge, skill, and character. A practice focuses on situated and relational knowledge—or knowledge gained from the context of the situation and interactions with the individuals present—and interpreting underdetermined and fluid situations that change over time and defy standardized rules and procedures. Challenges and concrete experiences help the nurse learn the stance of a good member-participant of nursing practice. Many of the notions of what constitutes good practice are not well articulated, and even when we see them described in these examples the *good* seems to be taken for granted. It is evident even without naming it.

Enthusiasm for nursing as a social good is a motivation for both students and teachers, and a "moral source" (Taylor, 2007) against fatigue and frustration. The passion of teachers and students was often quite evident in their social activism, for instance, working to decrease disparities in quality of or access to health care, or to improve care for the elderly or for inner-city school children. We found that nursing programs tend to address issues related to the health care system, and many though not all urge a critical perspective as part of formation. In our nine site visits, we found three schools where there was a conspicuous absence of a critical stance, where conformity and acceptance of the status quo in health care was more evident than curricular agendas of critique and reform of the existing health care system.

Most of the teachers and students we interviewed were consciously aware of status inequities and feminist issues seen in nursing being a predominantly white women's profession. A number of teachers, especially in the universities, were vehement in their calls for a more liberated, autonomous, and patient-centered approach to health care. A number of educators said that their motivation for teaching was to bring about change in the health care system:

> I came into teaching because I was just so upset about the way that psychiatric patients were treated on medical units. I did some acute-care hospital-psychiatric liaison work and saw a lot of ignorance and avoidance of patients with psychiatric diagnoses in acute care settings. They referred these patients to the psychiatric liaison nurse, saying, "Oh, but you just do something with them. We aren't going to ever talk to them. You take care of them. And when you can come down, *you* can do something, because we're just not able to go to that room anymore with them." Or, "They're crazy, and somebody has to sit with them." I mean, just really absurd things. And my goal really is that students will understand and get to like psychiatric patients, and

then when they get out into practice, that they will be able to model
that for other practitioners. Because I think it's pretty appalling what
exists in a lot of places . . . in most places.

Teachers often discussed the need for reform in the health care system,
including recognition and rewards for the responsibilities of professional
practice. They articulated how they hoped to improve nursing care and
health care institutions by teaching nursing students to be leaders and
change agents.

Master's-entry students, who are typically older with extensive life
experience and a strong academic background, were especially articulate
about the importance of addressing system-level problems in health care,
especially the disparities in health outcomes in the United States. Indeed,
the influx of these articulate students who aspire to change health care
on a systems level is also changing nursing schools, who must respond to
their demands for scholarship and activism. They are, in a sense, often "co-
creating" their educational experience. Formation of these students, many
with an advanced degree in another scholarly discipline, often challenges
teachers who are unused to such motivated, capable students demanding a
high level of scholarship from their teachers and voicing their disappoint-
ment if that demand is not met. Others see their students as an opportunity
to break free of old roles, focusing students on empowering them and rev-
olutionizing nursing so that it is focused more on health promotion, public
health, management of chronically ill patients, and improved care of the
elderly.

Faculty and students alike feel the tension of wanting to help institute positive, patient-centered changes while causing the least amount of
work and disruption possible at the clinical site. Helping clinical sites
adhere to best practices is an ongoing challenge for faculty and students
in many clinical sites. Students are seen as guests in their clinical setting, which impedes teachers and students from addressing instances of
poor practice. Student placements are limited and often tenuous. When
students and faculty are considered guests, students find being a legitimate member of a health team difficult. In the Carnegie-NSNA Survey
many students reported that they were unwelcome and disparaged in a
number of hospital settings. Faculty were also horrified by the treatment
many students received from staff nurses. This unwelcoming, dysfunctional behavior undercuts the ability of institutions to recruit students
as staff nurses. Solving this problem will require improving staffing levels
and work systems so that staff are not so overburdened. It will also require
culture change, and a new level of awareness of just how dangerous

to patient safety these dysfunctional communication patterns are in a hospital or any health care setting.

A reform agenda such as this is broad and far-reaching, and it calls for improved education of nurses as they attempt to change complex organizations and develop new health care policies and new health care delivery systems. Undergraduate students are presented with the dilemma of how to be such high-level reformers in their years of initial practice. These broad reform goals challenge the students to form an identity that is ill suited to the current health care system, while creating ambitious new models for how to be change agents in large bureaucratic settings where entry-level nurses have little social power. Drawing students' attention to the need for reform at a time when they have little hope of success at making changes creates a tension in the teaching and learning environment and the formation of nurses.

However, if professional styles of work organization are to be effective, professionals must learn how to influence organizational environments to support good practice, and administrators too must create environments where professionals can create self-improving practices (Sullivan, 2005). Organizational structures and processes that fit the functions and goals of good practice require ongoing design and development. For too long, nursing has not been at the institutional policy and decision-making tables. Both educators and students must approach their administrative and institutional responsibilities as nurses framed by the same notions of good that so admirably focus their work at the bedside. Teaching students to advocate for their patients and their profession at the institutional level is a necessary part of their formation, and schools of nursing must not abdicate this role. The end result will no doubt be better institutions as well as better-educated nurses.

Teaching students about institutional and bureaucratic systems and how to change them is yet another reason that it is essential to offer students engagement, whether in clinical situations or in the classroom, with the realities of care settings, complete with their real shortcomings as well as their positive supports for the practice. As this nurse educator explains, students' encounters with substandard practice settings can generate a sense of urgency for organizational and practice change:

> I had an opportunity to do a clinical with baccalaureate students in a less-than-ideal psychiatric setting, I'll put it that way. There were a lot of things going on that you don't want your students to model. And so, even though that was the case, it was a terrific learning experience, because we did get to talk about electric convulsive therapy as one of

the things. Also we were able to discuss and raise consciousness about the way that some of the nurses were interacting in a punitive way with the patients. The postclinical conferences were terrific because the students would come onto the unit and say, "I just saw this. Does this usually go on?" It was a great way to have a great teaching and learning conversation about improving practice.

It is not useful for students to internalize idealized, perfectionist versions of what institutions are or could be. They need to develop projects in actual clinical settings that reflect both evidence-based practice and exemplary nursing practice. Tools for influencing organizational and policy changes are essential, given the current state of health care institutions. Nurses are the ones most present and in a position closest to patients, and their advocacy for improving patient care can be powerful indeed. However, such positive change depends on knowledge and skills to redesign dangerous and outmoded systems and a unified effort to reduce communication barriers in hierarchical health care systems To create the level of change needed, partnerships between nurse educators and students in schools of nursing and nursing staff and administrators in service settings are essential. Regulatory bodies for health care institutions and all health care professions need to exert a unified effort at improved collaboration and communication. Each sector must enlarge its boundaries to include all nurses as members and participants in the larger good: effective nursing practice for the sake of a safer and healthier society.

PART FIVE

A CALL FOR RADICAL TRANSFORMATION

Many of my professors are wonderful and inspiring! And I know they earn next to nothing compared to what they could earn in the hospital so I have a lot respect for them! Nursing school is the most challenging thing I've done in my life but there are those moments with my patients when I'm reminded of why I decided to become a nurse and I feel it's worth it. I can't wait to become a nurse because I can't think of a greater career with more opportunities. I look forward to a career that I will love (most of the time) and the opportunity to provide a much needed service to society. And I feel that nursing is not just a job or even a career but part of who I am. I already feel that transformation. I'm starting to look at the world through a nurse's eyes.

As the challenge of her life, nursing school is a place where this student learns how to care for patients in a practice that she fully expects to love for many years and from teachers she deeply respects. Her comment speaks to nursing education at its best: situated teaching in the clinical setting, commitment to continuous improvement of care, pervasive concern on the part of educators for student formation, and shared dedication and zeal for becoming an excellent nurse.

Revealing an individual transformation no doubt, this student's comment also speaks to the radical transformation we call for in this book. We believe that the quality of nursing education is an urgent societal agenda. In our effort to increase the number nurses and nurse educators, we cannot be distracted from the need to redesign nursing education and close the practice-education gap for every nurse, whether new to the profession or a seasoned practitioner.

We invite the nursing community to join the call to action we gave in the Introduction. In Chapter Four, we outline four fundamental shifts in their approach to teaching that educators individually and programs collectively could make: (1) from a focus on decontextualized knowledge to an emphasis on teaching for a sense of salience, situated cognition, and action in clinical situations; (2) from a sharp separation of classroom and clinical teaching to integrative teaching in all settings; (3) from an emphasis on critical thinking to an emphasis on clinical reasoning and multiple ways of thinking that include critical thinking; and (4) from an emphasis on socialization and role taking to an emphasis on formation. We believe that in making these shifts, nursing education will achieve a deeper, more effective integration of the three apprenticeships.

In Parts Two, Three, and Four we offer the examples of Diane Pestolesi, Lisa Day, and Sarah Shannon, who over the course of their career have made these shifts in their thinking about teaching and attendant shifts in their expectations for student learning. Each has honed her craft of teaching through ongoing reflection and study of her teaching. All of these teachers took years to develop their approach to students, the curriculum, and learning. They draw directly from current practice and use their experience in the classroom effectively. They have realized that good nursing practice depends on their students' understanding of the patient's illness experience. Each guides her students to grasp the nature of the clinical situation and what the nurse's best and most appropriate responses to the whole situation are. They determine the educational gaps a student has, and they coach accordingly. They have high expectations for their students, regardless of the educational preparation of the student. They encourage their students to develop strong, active, and supportive learning communities. They like to be challenged by student questions they cannot readily answer. They are not threatened by questions or students arguing with them. Although we chose to focus on Pestolesi, Day, and Shannon, we observed many nurse educators who were similar in their approaches to their students and to teaching for a practice.

Good teaching in nursing requires that the teacher deeply understand good nursing practice, which Pestolesi, Day, and Shannon amply demonstrate. As Cossentino notes about learning to be an expert elementary school teacher:

> First is the importance of acknowledging that teaching expertise (like all expertise)... is constituted in particular cultural practices. Good practice is always connected to the "goods" of a given culture. Likewise, coherent practice may be viewed as a consequence of the intentional linkage between the hows, whys, and what fors of teaching. According to this model, coherence is located not in programming or policy, but in the act of teaching itself [Cossentino 2005, p. 239–240].

Although Cossentino refers to elementary school educators, she makes a point equally relevant for any level of education. Nursing schools often focus more on curricular structure, process, and content changes than on developing pedagogies that are relevant to nursing and helping faculty use them. Pestolesi, Day, and Shannon make clear for their students the hows, whys, and what fors of nursing. They have brought together knowledge, clinical reasoning, ethical comportment, and formation.

The paradigm cases of Pestolesi, Day, and Shannon make evident the reason educators, administrators, and students must leave behind the notion that "good" teachers are born or are successful only if the students are "good." They demonstrate the constant thought and attention needed for any professional practice: research, reflection, and learning that may lead to change. Just as nursing students learn clinical reasoning, not simply a set of skills that they use, so must teachers see their teaching as an integrated practice. The paradigm-case teachers approach their teaching as a practice in need of all the care and attention that any practice demands (Golde & Walker, 2006). In any field, excellent teaching requires critical reflection, continuous learning, the capacity to change and to question change, and ongoing development. In nursing, it also requires advanced knowledge of the practice.

Thus administrators of nursing education programs and the institutions where they are housed must understand, support, and finance the professional work for those who teach nursing students. So that educators can develop pedagogies and curricula that will support effective teaching and learning, our recommendations include support for faculty development within and across nursing programs and institutions as well as innovative ways to provide high-quality instruction in all areas of an integrated curriculum. Further, we call on national organizations to support efforts to improve curricula and pedagogy.

We realize that in many cases spheres of interest and responsibility overlap; regional and national chapters of professional organizations can play an important role in faculty development, for example, or articulated ADN-to-BSN programs. Moreover, there are resources and allies in other professions and disciplines. Nursing educators might not be the only ones on a community college or university campus who are trying to find more effective pedagogical approaches and engage in the scholarship of teaching and learning; working together with colleges in other professional programs or disciplines, nursing educators can better advocate for institutional resources. Likewise, teachers across the institution have much to teach and learn from one another. As nursing educators look beyond the confines of their programs and profession, we hope that they will discover and become engaged in the many regional and national efforts to improve postsecondary teaching and learning.

Improvement cannot be accomplished through curricular and pedagogical efforts alone: the changes that nursing education needs at the structural level are radical and require new approaches to policy. Practicing nurses, nursing administrators, preceptors, and nurse educators will need to act in concert with leaders of nursing organizations, regulatory bodies, state legislators, accreditors, and state boards of nursing to effect these important changes. Because the entire nursing community collectively holds the future of nursing, we close this book with a set of recommendations for individual educators, students, programs, institutions, professional organizations, and other stakeholders in the nation's health care system designed to preserve the strengths of nursing education and make much-needed changes.

To these ends, we offer a set of recommendations to the entire nursing education community. We expect and invite debate. We hope, however, for action.

13

IMPROVING NURSING EDUCATION AT THE PROGRAM LEVEL

THIS CHAPTER PRESENTS an agenda of recommendations to transform nursing education to meet today's needs. The recommendations presented are based on our findings and have been discussed in forums of nursing leaders in education, policy, research, and practice. Some of the recommendations are more controversial than others. Although not all in the nursing forums agreed with each one, we found strong support and interest for these recommendations and strong agreement on the problems identified.

The following recommendations fall into six general categories that speak to the need for change in nursing education: in nursing schools or programs, for student populations, in the ways student experience their education, in teaching the practice, in ways to enter practice, and for more coordinated national oversight. Several recommendations concern faculty development, which are best undertaken with a two-step approach. First, regional and national nursing organizations, graduate schools, and schools of nursing need to pool their resources to offer regional courses and workshops for educators to develop their teaching. At these meetings, nursing faculty can learn about new research findings. Second, faculty can then return to their individual institutions with knowledge about new pedagogies and new approaches to share with others.

To fulfill the professional promise nursing offers society nursing organizations and the service sector need to join nurse educators and students to improve nursing education before graduation and over the course of a nurse's career.

Entry and Pathways

1. *Come to agreement about a set of clinically relevant prerequisites.*
There is a pressing need to reevaluate the prerequisites for nursing education and address variation in quality and content. There is also a need in
many states to expand the number of available courses. We recommend
a national advisory group consisting of nursing faculty, clinicians, physicians, pharmacists, and expert science teachers agree on what prospective
students must know in the humanities, natural sciences, and social sciences
and how they are relevant to clinical practice before they begin their nursing programs. We expect that these prerequisites would be examined and
updated regularly—and that programs would honor them consistently.

We also recommend an agreement on relevant prerequisites for the
many students who are coming to nursing school with a baccalaureate or
advanced degree, many of whom have completed extensive coursework
in natural sciences, social sciences, and humanities. Although an increasing number of second-degree students are enrolled in all types of nursing
schools, nursing curricula have not changed to accommodate them. Accelerated second-degree baccalaureate programs are growing quickly, but for
reasons of affordability many second-degree students enroll in community
colleges—yet they have to spend three years completing the program. An
evaluation is needed to compare the learning needs of this new population of nursing students with students in generic baccalaureate programs.
The Fuld Foundation grant to the Duke University School of Nursing
is one example of such an evaluation that is still in its data collection
phase.

Given our findings on teaching and learning nursing knowledge and
science, we call into question the wisdom of not requiring more prerequisites or more coursework in science for RN-to-baccalaureate transition
programs. We recommend that the programs continue to be designed
for completion within two years. However, we recommend that these
programs develop and require relevant science courses tailored for the
individual RN-to-baccalaureate-degree student. Students who do not
place out of science entry examinations should be required to take these
courses.

2. *Require the BSN for entry to practice.* Unlike their colleague educators preparing lawyers, clergy, physicians, and engineers, nursing faculty
and preceptors have relatively little time to build a broad and deep
knowledge base and guide students in professional formation. Yet nursing requires a high degree of responsibility and judgment in high-risk,

underdetermined situations. Thus the baccalaureate degree in nursing should be the minimal educational level for entry into practice. We agree with the Association of American Colleges of Nursing, the American Nursing Association, and other leading nursing organizations that all nursing programs immediately move to baccalaureate degree or master's-level entry for nurses. We challenge the profession to come to swift agreement about the most effective way to transform the current diverse pathways into a unified whole.

3. *Develop local articulation programs to ensure a smooth, timely transition from the ADN to the BSN.* We recommend a redesign and reconfiguration of the roles of diploma and community colleges in nursing education. Currently, many ADN programs offer the baccalaureate degree in nursing, and more programs are in the planning stages. In general, we do not see the merit of this; it stretches the already overburdened community college mission and diminishes its capacity and role in opening access to educational paths. What was meant to constitute a swift entry to practice has resulted in a logjam, and students are not moving on to the BSN in appreciable numbers. We urge local and regional consortiums, on the order of the Oregon Consortium for Nursing Education, to create a seamless transition from the ADN program to the BSN—and beyond.

4. *Develop more ADN-to-MSN programs.* We recommend increasing the number of ADN-to-MSN programs. Orsolini-Hain (2008) found that few ADN students felt motivated to return to school for a baccalaureate degree because the degree would not significantly influence their job capacities and functions. We believe that ADN-to-MSN programs would appeal to practicing ADNs and give them a realistic incentive to return to school for better job opportunities and salaries. Another benefit of this action would be growth of the applicant pool for doctoral study and enlargement of the faculty pipeline.

Student Population

5. *Recruit a more diverse faculty and student body.* We note that African Americans, Hispanic Americans, Asian Americans, and American Indians are underrepresented in nursing. As a profession nursing remains far from being as diverse as the populations it serves. Yet to practice, nurses must be attuned to the diversity of concerns, attitudes, and values that patients and their families bring to bear on their health. This attunement comes in part from a diverse profession. Underrepresented minorities are also are more likely than others to pursue the baccalaureate or a higher degree

in nursing (AACN, 2008) and thus be ready for graduate school, which could lead to a more diverse nursing faculty. Local, regional, and national efforts to recruit more diverse students and faculty are needed. We note that schools and health care organizations offer outreach and pipeline programs for high school students, and we commend these programs and recommend that they be strengthened through continued financial support and recruitment and retention infrastructures. It is essential that health care institutions increase their commitment to supporting education as well as their diversity. Such commitment could be shown through growth in incentives for minority nurses to become nurse educators, including more scholarships for minority nurses and active recruitment for minority nurses to pursue graduate education.

6. *Provide more financial aid, whether from public or private sources, for all students, at all levels.* Many health care organizations have created programs to make loans that are reduced or forgiven if the graduate works for the organization. We commend these efforts and recommend more focused attention by federal, state, and local authorities to support the education of nurses. In addition, every health science education center could add fellowships to the annual campaign in order to immediately address the shortfall in funding for nursing and medical education. In the context of the acute nursing shortage, new opportunities exist to encourage state governments to offer more entitlements for nursing scholarships through education taxes imposed on new health care facility extensions.

The Student Experience

7. *Introduce prenursing students to nursing early in their education.* Nursing programs are short, yet the formation of nurses is complex. Programs should take the earliest opportunity to introduce students to the profession. We note that BSN programs could bring students into the nursing curriculum earlier, before the junior year. For example, first-year (that is, freshman) students who intend to be nurses might take a seminar on nursing. We also recommend that they begin taking prerequisites for clinical courses during the first two years of college. The school would also need to offer summer courses to accommodate students who transfer or do not decide on their nursing major until the sophomore year. However, the advantage of beginning to use and integrate knowledge early from prerequisite science and humanities and the additional time for formation produce a strong rationale for an earlier start to nursing courses.

8. *Broaden the clinical experience.* Although the amounts vary by type of program, much of a nursing student's clinical time in school is focused on acute-care hospital practice. However, more than 50 percent of nurses now work outside the hospital setting. With an aging population, more nurses will be needed for staffing and upgrading the quality of long-term institutional and home care. Likewise, community health care and school nursing have become more important as more of the population is underinsured or uninsured. Placements in such settings can have the added benefit of making the profession visible to a broader population of prospective students. Increasing the variety of clinical settings would also address a common student complaint: that clinical schedules are not announced well in advance and often involve long student commute times to clinical placements and variable and unpredictable hours that make it difficult to coordinate school, work, and family responsibilities. Although it is difficult for school administrators to predict clinical site availability, every effort must be made to set student schedules as far in advance as possible. We recommend flexibility wherever possible in helping students find clinical sites and schedules that accommodate their home and work life.

9. *Preserve postclinical conferences and small patient-care assignments.* When students have the opportunity to reflect on their clinical experiences, the power of experiential learning increases. Students need time to reflect on their care of patients, and the postclinical conference is an ideal time for that reflection. We observed many conferences focused on continuous improvement of care provided. As they continued the situated coaching that they had used while the students were with their patients, the teachers guided the students in developing a sense of salience, using knowledge in clinical situations and taking action steps related to knowledge and skills.

We noted, also, that students are better able to reflect on their practice if they care for only one or two patients at a time. We found that the patient assignments given to students strongly influenced their ability to reason on behalf of and solve problems with their patients. Students also highly valued their smaller patient-care assignments of one or two patients. They explained that they could get to know their patients, develop their relational and communication skills, and increase their understanding of the patient's experience.

Even so, pressure from employers mounts, and many programs operate on an untested assumption that handling larger patient care loads will make the students more efficient on graduation. We believe that larger patient-care assignments, and the attendant cut in time for learning and reflection, will contribute to gaps in the student's understanding of the nurse-patient relationship and communication. Moreover, few schools have clinical curricula that allow students to follow patients and families across time and institutional settings. Students thus focus on acute and episodic assignments in hospital settings, caring for patients over one or two days.

We recommend small patient-care assignments of one to two patients at the start of each new clinical rotation. In addition to the experience of providing total patient care, we recommend that students have the opportunity in each specialty to work with nurses with such clinical specialties as infection control, quality and safety improvement, and discharge planning.

10. *Develop pedagogies that keep students focused on the patient's experience.* We recommend teaching medical pathology and disease mechanisms in direct association with patients' illness experiences, psychosocial aspects of illness, patient and family coping, and teaching of self-care.

Attendant to this approach would be support for teachers to learn to scaffold their course around patient care. Examples of pedagogies are simulation exercises, the unfolding cases that Lisa Day uses in her class, narrative structures for making a case, and interviews of patients in class. Whether during a simulation nurse educators use expensive mannequins, or simply a few props to mimic a clinical situation, they have the luxury of being able to start and stop it. They can then pose questions to students, ask them to think about clinical puzzles, or discuss rationales for treatment in more detail than is appropriate while caring for patients. By coaching students to focus on actual patients in specific situations, teachers give students the opportunity to rehearse aloud or in writing the appropriate care of communities and patients and their families. It is important to keep in mind though that the ability to stop and start the exercise is at odds with actual clinical situations. In short, it can be difficult for students to be fully engaged when a simulation stops and starts. It can also be difficult for many to engage in solving clinical puzzles with a mannequin. We recommend that during simulation exercises, as Lisa Day does, the nurse educator return often to the experience of the patient and the patient's responses to therapies.

Further, we recommend that regional and national resources be made available for developing effective and sophisticated clinical simulation exercises that are designed to help students integrate knowledge, skilled know-how, and ethical comportment. One aim of integrative teaching is to foster students' grasp of practice concerns that allow them to develop clinical imagination or the ability to envision how they would approach patients and their families and care for them.

11. *Vary the means of assessing student performance.* How learning is assessed sends a powerful message about what the profession believes to be important. We found that nursing education could significantly improve assessment of student learning, particularly clinical performance and knowledge use; however, educators must be supported in learning new assessment strategies. We found too few means of assessing the student knowledge and skill acquisition necessary for practice, and we worry that there is too much focus on strategies to answer multiple-choice questions on exams, such as the NCLEX-RN. We saw many lost opportunities for assessing student knowledge and skill acquisition. Clinical teachers informally assess students' skilled know-how in the context of patient care, but too often their formal assessment of students is through written clinical assignments, such as care plans, which are poor proxies for how a student might perform in a clinical situation. Observation for the purpose of assessing student performance in the clinical setting should be formative, deliberate, and ongoing.

We recommend that educators use varied assessments—both formative and summative—for clinical performance, and conduct them in different settings, including simulation exercises, skills laboratories, classrooms with actor patients, and directly in the clinical setting. Indicators of clinical performance should include, for example, how well students are able to set priorities in a clinical situation, develop a rationale for patient care, or respond to changes in patients. Students should also be assessed on their skills of clinical reasoning and their ability to solve clinical puzzles.

12. *Promote and support learning the skills of inquiry and research.* We recommend, for example, that faculty require students to try to follow through on the care of their patients. By examining discharge outcomes, students would discover the consequences of their patient care, as well as learn about the hospital trajectory of patients and discharge planning for every patient. We also recommend that students be expected to learn research skills and access the nursing literature. Students should learn to search relevant research and patient population-based evidence for care of their patients before and after their clinical assignment. In addition, we recommend that all students be equipped with electronic data management equipment, such as handheld personal data assistants, to help them access just-in-time information.

13. *Redesign the ethics curricula.* Nursing students need to learn about critical ethics and dilemma ethics, but also everyday ethical comportment related to relational or care ethics. Students must learn everyday ethical comportment and the notions of good central to the profession. Student nurses need to learn the ethics of care and responsibility, the ethos of self-care in the profession, skills of involvement, and clinical reasoning. Students need to be able to reflect on and articulate their everyday ethical concerns, and not limit their understanding to ethical breakdowns and dilemmas.

In addition, we recommend nurse educators focus on everyday ethical comportment. Narrative pedagogies, such as experience-based narratives of practice situations, journals, or debriefing and reflection on practice, are also effective ways to uncover and articulate everyday ethical comportment and notions of good central to nursing practice.

14. *Support students in becoming agents of change.* Today's students can become powerful leaders ready to influence the larger political and public arenas for improved health care systems. They will need to learn strategies to change organizations, theories of organizational development, and policy making in order to be prepared to meet the reform challenges in practice settings.

We recommend that all levels of nursing education, including school-to-work transition and continuing nursing education programs, prepare students for the complex bureaucratic settings where they will practice, continue to learn, and teach. Students need practical strategies for how to incorporate evidence-based practice and best practices for patient safety into their particular organizational setting. Students also need increased focus on knowledge and skills of critical reflection about the health care system that help them conceive of organizational change and health care policy development.

Teaching

15. *Fully support ongoing faculty development for all who educate student nurses.* As Shulman and others (Boyer, 1990; Huber & Hutchings, 2005; Shulman & Wilson, 2004) have pointed out, there are few mechanisms for teachers to document their learning, critically examine their practices, and advance the quality of work in their field. Nursing is no exception. Educators report that they do not have enough time or opportunity to reflect on their teaching or the quality of student learning. The combination of lack of basic teacher preparation in graduate

nursing schools and limited faculty development conspires to thwart effective teaching and learning.

Indeed, the current lack of focus on teaching is a central challenge to elevating the quality and effectiveness of nursing education. As do teachers in other professions, teachers of nursing tend to carry out their work in isolation from their colleagues in either the classroom or the clinical setting; teaching is rarely reviewed or evaluated constructively by peers, and those who develop innovative and effective approaches to teaching rarely build on the work of others. Moreover, teachers of nursing must teach for a practice while staying current in a field that is rapidly growing and changing. We noted very little effort to make teaching practices public, accessible, and therefore available for study and improvement.

We recommend that nursing educators be fully supported in reflecting on and improving their teaching practice. At the most basic level, educators should be supported in investigating the goals and outcomes of teaching, and evaluating their choice of teaching strategies, starting with such basic questions as, What kinds of responses are expected from students during a classroom session? What kinds of imaginative access to the practice does the class provide? What is the level of information presented and represented in the exchange of questions and answers between students and teachers? What is the extent of integration between classroom and clinical education? In the recommendations that follow in this section, we suggest some particular areas of faculty development for specific teaching strategies and learning outcomes.

We recommend rich faculty development opportunities at the local, regional, and national levels. Faculty development is the responsibility of individual teachers, programs, institutions, AACN, NLN, the state boards of nursing, and professional societies. These groups could convene to address these aims:

○ Enhance the practice of teaching in the profession.

○ Improve promotion and faculty development incentives and rewards for good teaching.

○ Develop curricula and pedagogies that foster lifelong learning and clinical inquiry skills in student nurses.

Within these areas, there is wide scope to develop research programs focused on pedagogies for nursing. Research questions could include:

○ What are styles and patterns of highly successful, and unsuccessful, approaches to teaching and learning for good nursing practice?

○ What kinds of projects or educational tools (such as unfolding cases, simulations) have the most significant impact on student learning?

○ What kinds of information, resources, and models are needed to ensure that efforts to promote the scholarship of teaching have an impact beyond the individual participants involved?

○ How do teachers learn and demonstrate exemplary teaching for a sense of salience at each level of nursing education?

○ What are successful strategies of integration of classroom and clinical teaching and learning of nursing, natural sciences, social sciences, and humanities?

○ What knowledge from cross-professional education could be effectively imported and adapted for nursing education?

To support the scholarship of teaching and learning will require increased support on the part of schools, federal and state governments, and philanthropies. Innovative funding strategies are needed; the California Work Force Team on Nursing is considering an increase in licensing fees and earmarking this money for nursing education. Other strategies of sustainable funding structured into state budgets as well as nurse employer budgets, and many more new funding initiatives in nursing education, will be needed. The California Work Force Team is also participating in the National Coalition Project on Nursing to explore the possibility of taxing the hospitals that are developing new patient care bed capacities to help fund the education of the new nurses required for these units. Another possible source of funds for nursing education might be taxes on Medicare or other national health care plans.

16. *Include teacher education courses in master's and doctoral programs.* To be responsible stewards of the discipline (Golde & Walker, 2006; Walker et al., 2008), all graduate nursing programs need to support the study of pedagogies designed and evaluated for nursing education. We recommend that all master's and doctoral programs include teacher education courses and experience that better prepare future nursing faculty for teaching. An important caveat is that master's programs with a nursing education major must also ensure advanced clinical practice preparation for future teachers.

17. *Foster opportunities for educators to learn how to teach students to reflect on their practice.* Programs and professional organizations must support educators in learning how to create a safe climate for students to reflect on their learning experiences, both successes and mistakes.

We suggest, for example, local, regional, and national conferences on pedagogies of reflection such as student-generated accounts of learning from their experiences with patients and families or ways of guiding students in discussion of their strengths and errors in patient care and the strengths and mistakes of other health care team members. Other strategies might include journals and small group discussions like those in postclinical conferences, where students give first-person accounts of their clinical learning experiences. These discussions are opportunities for students to reflect as they discuss the strengths and mistakes of other health care team members. We also urge faculty to use vignettes from their clinical practice and invite former patients to class discuss their experiences of illness and care.

To guide discussions about practice breakdown or errors, we suggest educators enrich courses on dilemma-based ethics and bioethics with attention to everyday notions of good practice and relational ethics.

18. *Support faculty in learning how to coach*. Rich and situated coaching is routinely part of teaching in the clinical setting, and we recommend that such coaching on practical clinical reasoning be extended to the classroom, so that students are asked to think and solve problems in situations that more closely resemble what they will encounter when they take care of patients. We recommend that all teachers, whether in the classroom or a clinical setting, use coaching and ask questions about a particular situation such as, "Why are you giving that medication at this time?" "in order to accomplish what?" and "for the sake of what concern?"

19. *Support educators in learning how to use narrative pedagogies*. Learning to think like a nurse involves developing skill with narrative structures and narrative thinking; an understanding of the clinical situation; the ability to find science-based answers to pathophysiology, therapies, signs and symptoms; and the relational and communication skills of listening to and clarifying patient and family concerns. Because injuries and illness occur in the context of a person's life, the nurse must formulate a narrative of the patient's immediate clinical history, his concerns, and even an account of his life and lifeworld. Reasoning across time involves the ability to construct a sensible story of immediate events, their sequence, and their consequences, in terms of illness trajectories and life concerns.

Programs and professional organizations should support educators in learning how to use narrative pedagogies in the classroom and skills labs. Narrative pedagogies are among the best teaching strategies we observed, and they are effective in developing students' sense of salience, clinical reasoning, and clinical judgment. Such narrative pedagogies include student journals, simulation, or patient interviews during class time. They are also important for developing clinical imagination, by helping students imagine their actions or approaches to the care of patient populations, communities, patients, and families.

20. *Provide faculty with resources to stay clinically current.* Many teachers find ways to stay current in their clinical specialty. Yet even teachers who are currently engaged in practice cannot reasonably expect to have current clinical knowledge and practices in every area of a clinically focused course. We found, however, that some classroom teachers have not been in practice for many years. In the worst cases, students complained that their classroom teachers were neither prepared to be teachers nor up-to-date in their understanding of current clinical practice.

Faculty enrichment and development might take the form of inviting expert clinical nurse specialists or other specialists to prepare classroom teachers with the most current knowledge about a particular clinical practice area. School administrators might invite expert clinical nurse specialists or other specialists to impart up-to-date knowledge about a clinical practice area. Expert educators as well as discipline-specific educators could be recruited to assist in these faculty development efforts.

Likewise, guest lecturers with specialized, advanced clinical knowledge offering depth and currency in clinical practice and research could be invited into the classroom. However, we caution that such learning sessions need careful design, tailoring, and integration. For continuity and coherence, the faculty of record must actively integrate and coordinate any guest lectures with ongoing teaching and learning in the class. Otherwise, the course loses coherence and becomes a series of classes, or worse disconnected lectures, rather than an integrated whole.

Partnerships with clinical facilities would help in identifying outstanding clinical scholar-practitioners who could augment and enrich classroom exploration of advanced patient care in specific clinical topics. This might take the form of collaboration of educators with experts in relevant clinical fields.

21. *Improve the work environment for staff nurses, and support them in learning to teach.* Our observations and student reports noted that clinical placements are often overcrowded. Students also reported they experienced uncivil, if not hostile, behavior from staff nurses. We urge health care employers to improve the work environment for nurses, including patient and nurse safety and workload. In particular, we recommend

zero tolerance for uncivil behavior toward any member of the health care team, including student nurses and other health care professionals in training.

At the same time, providing opportunities for staff nurses to learn to teach would decrease the widely varying quality of teaching and coaching by staff nurses. Although called "partnering staff nurse teachers," these members of the teaching team often receive no guidance in teaching, much less the clinical objectives for the particular course. We recommend employers create ongoing opportunities for nurses in practice settings to learn how to teach and coach students.

22. *Address the faculty shortage.* According to AACN's 2003–04 report *Enrollment and Graduations in Baccalaureate and Graduate Programs in Nursing*, U.S. schools of nursing turned away 15,944 applicants qualified to participate in entry-level baccalaureate programs. The report cited insufficient faculty, clinical sites, classroom space, and clinical preceptors, along with budget constraints. At the same time, faculty report a perceived higher workload than what faces their campus colleagues in other programs. Moreover, faculty salaries are considerably lower than salaries for clinical positions or for teaching in other disciplines.

Efforts to recruit students into graduate programs that could lead to teaching positions will be futile unless faculty salaries are increased and brought into line with clinical salaries and those for teaching positions in other disciplines. Health care organizations and nursing schools (and their institutions) must come into agreement about flexible practice schedules and salaries.

Many schools of nursing offer their faculty access to centralized teaching and learning resources that adequately meet the needs of nursing faculty. However, for those whose needs are not met, we recommend schools and national nursing organizations collaborate to develop programs that help nursing faculty teach with faculty from other disciplines. We propose schools recruit or collaborate with faculty who are not nurses but who are prepared at the doctoral level in science, social science, or humanities. These specialists from other disciplines must be committed to teaching pre-licensure nursing students and furthering knowledge in nursing. After finishing their doctoral work, they must be prepared by nurse educators to teach for nursing practice, whether through online courses or extended and in-depth conferences devoted to the scholarship of teaching and learning for professional practice. This recommendation seeks to enrich nursing education and ease the burden of teaching that is imposed on personnel-strapped programs. Hiring colleagues from other disciplines would have the added benefit of increasing interdisciplinary approaches to nursing and nursing education. We further recommend that nurse educators co-teach with these colleagues so that they too have opportunities to learn.

Entry to Practice

23. *Develop clinical residencies for all new graduates.* Improving prelicensure nursing education is an important and necessary step in addressing the practice-education gap. The extent and nature of learning that students need cannot be deferred to postgraduate clinical residencies. Indeed, it is wrong-headed to allow the responsibility for what should be taught in prelicensure education to pass to postgraduation residency programs. However, we recommend that all graduates be required to complete a one-year residency program focused on one clinical area of specialization so that the graduate has the opportunity to develop in-depth knowledge in that area. During these residencies, mentors can teach local styles of practice and particular innovations characteristic of all health care settings. We also recommend evaluation that identifies practice-educational gaps; such evaluation should include patient outcomes. To offset the costs of these programs, we recommend lower entry-level salaries for the residency year.

24. *Change the requirements for licensure.* Although our study focused on education for entry to practice, our findings speak to the redesign of nursing education as a whole. Nurses in all programs are currently undereducated for current nursing practice demands. In addition to answering the serious problem of undereducation of nurses, we recommend that boards of registered nurses require graduates who pass the NCLEX-RN after 2012 must earn a master's degree within ten years.

National Oversight

25. *Require performance assessments for licensure.* Currently, the service sector and educators agree that improved assessment of competencies is necessary for maintaining nursing licenses. State boards of nursing in the United States (NCSBN, 2005) and accrediting bodies in Canada (Canadian Nurses' Association [CNA], no date) as well citizen's groups such

as the Citizen Advocacy Center (Swankin, LeBuhn, & Morrison, 2006) are calling for better evaluation of continuing competency of nurses. All these groups maintain that taking continuing education courses does not lend sufficient evidence of continuing competence for practicing nurses (Ironside, 2008; Tilley, 2008). Nursing students should be exposed to such competency evaluations during their undergraduate programs in order to prepare them for continuing competency clinical performance exams that are likely to be a part of their professional life. Expanding the types of evaluation strategies, and especially including performance exams, will increase the validity of nursing school programs of study to predict successful and safe practice of their graduate nurses.

We recommend the National Council for State Boards of Nursing develop a new set of student performance assessments, with three national examinations of performance. This set of performance assessments should start during the beginning of the last year of nursing school with the first performance examination. The next should be given at the same time the student sits for the NCLEX-RN examination and the last at the end of a one-year postlicensure residency. These examinations could be given in simulation laboratories or with trained patient actors.

26. *Cooperate on accreditation.* We recommend that the separate agencies for accreditation—accrediting arms of NLN and AACN—come together to collaborate. As ADN programs affiliate with BSN programs, the accrediting agencies will need to cooperate more closely to ensure that articulation efforts are successful. In collaboration with other professional organizations and nursing administrators, and with help from faculty and preceptors, both agencies will need to come to agree on student outcomes, articulation of ADN, BSN, and MSN programs, and student transitions. They should also set meaningful standards for ongoing faculty development to ensure that educators are appropriately supported in their professional practice of teaching.

Another area where the accrediting agencies must cooperate is interdisciplinary education. We found almost no interdisciplinary learning or practice opportunities for students. Most nursing schools endorse interdisciplinary teaching and learning as a worthy goal, and some schools promote volunteer clinical opportunities for students, but we saw no interdisciplinary coursework, classes, or teaching in the clinical setting. Learning to practice in an interdisciplinary setting can help students work more effectively on a health care team as well as better integrate knowledge, skilled know-how, and ethical comportment in practice. Finally, the agencies should work together to systematically review current demands for knowledge and skill as well as scan for future trends for nursing practice.

Taken together, the Carnegie Foundation studies on professional education point to a new moral vision for the professions, where professional responsibility, accountability, and ethical comportment constitute a fulcrum for their identity and action. Now the nursing profession must unite and act to regain excellence in nursing education. This will take bold action on the part of educators, but our society and nurses themselves deserve nothing less.

METHODS FOR THE CARNEGIE NATIONAL NURSING EDUCATION STUDY

THE NURSING STUDY is one in the series of studies known as the Preparation for the Professions Program, supported by the Carnegie Foundation for the Advancement of Teaching. The series comprises separate studies of professional education in law, clergy, engineering, medicine, and nursing. The purpose of the series is to determine the signature pedagogies of professional education, compare and contrast educational methods, and determine how to educate for both competence and integrity, how to educate for professional judgment, and how to teach complex skills. As it is embedded in this series of studies, the methods and interview questions for the Carnegie Foundation National Nursing Education Study were based on the previous completed studies. However, as was the case with each study, the nursing study included variations in questions to address pedagogical concerns and content, which are discipline-specific.

The nursing study compares and evaluates nine schools of nursing. In keeping with the larger Carnegie Preparation for the Professions Program, three dimensions of professional education and formation are examined: (1) learning of theory and scientific methods, (2) the mastery of skillful practice, (3) the formation of professional identity and agency. All three areas—skillful ethical comportment, good clinical judgment, and use of the best scientific knowledge—must be integrated in the identity and actions of the professional nurse. Therefore, they are studied separately and as a whole.

The general study design is ethnographic, interpretive, and evaluative. The data collection strategies included: classroom observation, a syllabus interview, and student and faculty interview for two selected major courses in the curriculum. In addition there are faculty interviews, administrative interviews, preceptor interviews, individual student interviews, student focus groups, and finally observation of students engaged in clinical practice. This study also uses three Web-based surveys of nursing faculty and nursing students to confirm/disconfirm our site visit findings. The surveys are conducted in collaboration with the National League for Nursing, the American Association of Colleges of Nursing, and the National Student Nurses' Association.

Description of the Nine Site Visits

The first phase of the Carnegie Foundation National Carnegie Education Study was to conduct nine site visits to entry-level nursing programs in the United States and one RN-to-BSN program. The programs, selected in geographically diverse areas, were one diploma, two associate degree, three traditional baccalaureate degree, two fast-track baccalaureate degree, one master's entry-level, and one RN-to-BSN. There were five criteria for selecting schools:

1. The school had an excellent reputation for teaching and learning.
2. The prelicensure programs had a high state board examination pass rate.
3. The schools were recommended by either an accrediting body or a state board of education.
4. Additional consideration was given to achieving a geographic sampling, and accommodating a school's academic calendar.
5. A decision was made to study an associate degree program in California; both the researchers and the nursing associations had heard that a two-year, associate degree program in California could take as long as four to five years to complete because of the prerequisites.

The goal was to focus on the best practices of teaching rather than looking for deficits or judging the programs against prespecified criteria. The Carnegie Foundation requested that we visit at least two of the same schools as were found in the Medical Education Study. The University of California, San Francisco, and the University of Washington in Seattle were determined to be schools visited jointly by the nursing and medicine teams. Both of these schools met our criteria for excellence because they are consistently ranked the number one and number two nursing schools in the country. Additional schools were chosen through collaboration with the Tri-Council of Nursing, made up of the American Association of Colleges of Nursing and Commission on Collegiate Nursing Education, the American Nurses Association, the American Organization of Nurse Executives, and the National League for Nursing and National League for Nursing Accrediting Commission; and with the National Council of State Boards of Nursing. All of these organizations agreed to advise on relevant studies of nursing education already conducted by the professional societies, and to assist with developing policy implications and implementing findings from the study.

The nine schools selected were first contacted by phone by the principal investigator. This was followed up with an explanatory letter. All of the schools agreed to participate in the study. Each school received feedback at the end of the visit regarding what had been learned from other sites and selected observations about best practices in the school. Participating schools were invited to attend an invitational conference at the conclusion of the data collection and analysis to present findings.

Human subjects approval was obtained from the Committee on Human Subjects Review at the University of California, San Francisco, and from the Institutional Review Board at the Carnegie Foundation after an invitation to participate was accepted by each of the participating schools. We also sought and received approval from the Institutional Review Board of Samuel Merritt College in Oakland, California. Samuel Merritt College was to be our original pilot site.

Design of the Site Visit Interview Instruments

Data Sources and Collection

Questions were developed that were comparable to the questions and interview protocols from the Preparation for the Professions studies of law, engineering, and clergy. Nineteen protocols with preformulated and nursing-specific questions were used for the nursing study as interview guides.

Site visits were held in the winter, spring, summer, and fall of 2005 over a ten-month period. Five researchers assigned to the project along with senior scholars from the Carnegie Foundation conducted the site visits. A typical site visit was preceded by approximately five to seven telephone interviews with key administrators and faculty of the syllabus courses. In some cases, course materials such as a course syllabus were made available to the team before the site visit or phone interview. The site visit was approximately three days long and was made up of observations, interviews, and focus group discussions.

The site visit was structured broadly by the Carnegie research team, and then specific scheduling was done at the campus level. A typical basic schedule consisted of:

- An orientation and overview meeting
- Classroom observations
- Student focus groups, including interviews with students who were participants in the syllabus course observed and narrative interviews of students getting ready to graduate from the program
- Clinical and didactic faculty focus groups
- Clinical site observations
- Observations of postclinical conferences
- A closure meeting with faculty

Team members wrote extensive field notes using a common guide on each campus and site visit. In addition, a history and description of each school and its curriculum were obtained from the school's Website prior to the site visit. Clinical observations required us to follow the students, or observe groups of students working together, with their instructor or working with a patient. Informal interviews conducted away from the patient care setting asked students about their experience. Otherwise, observations and informal interviews were captured in extensive field notes written by the observer.

Clinical observations were held at the student clinical placement sites. We observed individual students, students and their instructors, or students with patients. During these observations, field notes were taken. Classroom observations were scheduled during the site visit and typically attended by two or more of the researchers, including the researcher who had conducted the interview of the teacher prior to or after the site visit. Using the appropriate protocol for the classroom observation as a guide, each researcher made extensive field notes. Field notes and observations were discussed in team debriefings to compare and validate observations. Where possible, the classes were attended by three or four researchers so that rich and comparative observation and assessments could be made.

Soniclear Recorder Pro, a computer program that digitally records voices, was used in small group interviews, and handheld digital recorders were used for field notes as well as informal interviews with students in their clinical placements. With the advance consent of the interviewee, telephone interviews were recorded using a phone tap device and Soni-clear Recorder Pro equipment. The interviews were then transferred onto the Carnegie Foundation secured shared drive using a computer uploading procedure. The project administrative assistant then sent the interviews out for transcription. A paid transcriptionist prepared interview materials and returned them to the Carnegie Foundation's secure shared drive in written format, where they were accessible only to the entire research team. All transcripts were examined for accuracy by the project assistant, comparing the tape recorded interviews with the transcribed text.

Interpretation of the Data

Indexing the Data: Developing Codes

A list of codes developed from the interviews of 586 students, faculty, and administrators was developed over a five-month period. Initially, our team reviewed the same interviews and discussed our understandings and interpretations of specific portions of text and suggested themes. The team settled on twenty-two main codes, with subtheme categories under each main code. The data were coded and entered into the qualitative software management tool NVivo. Analysis of all the qualitative data then proceeded inductively from this indexed data.

Design of the Surveys

Data Sources and Collection

Starting from analysis of the site visit data, the researchers developed two surveys for faculty and one for students with questions on teaching and learning. The survey questions were designed to help the researchers confirm or disconfirm the site visit findings. The surveys were piloted on a small group of local educators and students. The three surveys are conducted in collaboration with the National League for Nursing, the American Association of Colleges of Nursing, and the National Student Nurses' Association. The surveys were Web-based, with links to the surveys sent to all members of each organization. The National Student Nurses' Association–Carnegie Foundation and the American Association of Colleges of Nursing–Carnegie Foundation surveys were housed on Survey Monkey, a company that hosts Web-based surveys. The National League for Nursing–Carnegie Foundation survey was hosted by the organization.

Table 1.1 Number of Surveys Returned

Organizations Collaborating with the Carnegie Foundation	Number of Surveys Returned
AACN (faculty)	123
NLN (faculty)	8,486
NSNA (student)	1,648

Interpretation of the Data

Indexing the Data: Developing Codes

All the qualitative survey data were entered into the qualitative software data analysis tool NVivo. A thematic analysis was done in order to answer each question in each major line of inquiry: curriculum, pedagogies, learning, and assessment. All the answers to the open-ended questions on the two Web-based surveys were entered into NVivo and a thematic analysis was conducted on the categories of curriculum, pedagogies, learning, and assessment.

Identifying Paradigm Cases

A number of excellent teachers were selected as potential paradigm cases to illustrate exemplary integrative teaching in nursing. We settled on three who were particularly articulate about their change as teacher over time, their reflection on and articulation about their teaching, and finally because each was innovative and had high student evaluations. Each paradigm teacher's articulation of her teaching matched the students' understanding of what they learned from the teacher.

Writing Up the Findings

Writing and rewriting the findings in qualitative research is essential to the intellectual and scholarly work of this form of research. In the writing, we integrated findings from the three national surveys and site visits (see Table 1.2). The multiple reviews with Anne Colby, William Sullivan, and Lee Shulman helped us be clearer in our descriptions and articulation of the nature of the domain-specific teaching in nursing. Finally, we have written up the findings so that the reader can participate in the

Table 1.2   Index of Research Site Visit Protocols

A	Consent Forms
1	Protocol for School Document Analysis
2	Protocol for Conversation/Interview with Executive Officer/Dean
3	Academic Dean Interview
4	Discussion Guide with Program Directors
5	Admissions Officer Interview
6	Interview for Student Services Representative
7	Discussion Guide with Clinical Preceptors
8	Protocol for Faculty Focus Group
9	Syllabus Interview Letter
10	Syllabus Interview
11	Classroom Visit, Observation Protocol
12	Protocol for Sophomore Student Focus Group Linked with Pivotal Course
13	Protocol for Senior Student Focus Group Linked with Pivotal Course
14	Protocol for Narrative Senior Student Focus Group
15	Student Focus Group Participant Background Questionnaire
16	Faculty Focus Group Participant Background Questionnaire
17	Exit Interview
18	Reflections on Site Visit

consensual validation of our interpretations. To this end, we include many interview excerpts in the book to give the reader the chance to evaluate our interpretations.

REFERENCES

Aiken, L. H., Clarke, S. P., & Sloane, D. M. (2002). Hospital Staffing, Organization, and Quality of Care: Cross-National Findings. *International Journal for Quality in Health Care, 14*(1), 5–13.

Aiken, L. H., Clarke, S. P., Sloane, D. M., Sochalski, J., & Silber, J. H. (2002). Hospital Nurse Staffing and Patient Mortality, Nurse Burnout, and Job Dissatisfaction. *Journal of the American Medical Association, 288*(16), 1987–1993.

American Association of Colleges of Nursing. (2007a). *Annual State of the Schools.* Washington, DC: American Association of Colleges of Nursing.

American Association of Colleges of Nursing. (2007b). *FY 2008 Recommendation: Increase Funding for Title VIII Nursing Workforce Development Programs.* Retrieved January 27, 2008, from http://www.aacn.nche.edu/government/pdf/08TitleVIIIFS.pdf.

American Association of Colleges of Nursing. (2007c). *2006–2007 Salaries of Instructional and Administrative Nursing Faculty in Baccalaureate and Graduate Programs in Nursing.* Washington, DC: American Association of Colleges of Nursing.

American Association of Colleges of Nursing. (2008). *2007–2008 Enrollment and Graduations in Baccalaureate and Graduate Programs in Nursing.* Washington, DC: American Association of Colleges of Nursing.

American Hospital Association. (2007). *The 2007 State of America's Hospitals: Taking the Pulse, Findings from the 2007 AHA Survey of Hospital Leaders.* Chicago: American Hospital Association.

American Nurses Association [ANA] Gallup Poll (2008). Nurses Voted Most Trusted Profession. http://www.nursingworld.org/FunctionalMenuCategories/MediaResources/PressReleases/2008PR/Nurses-Most-Trusted.aspx.

American Organization of Nurse Executives. (2005). *BSN-Level Nursing Education Resources.* Retrieved June 1, 2008, from http://www.aone.org/aone/resource/practiceandeducation.html.

Arford, P. H. (2005). Nurse-Physician Communication: An Organizational Accountability. *Nursing Economics, 23*(2), 72–77.

Auerbach, D. I., Buerhaus, P. I., & Staiger, D. O. (2007). Better Late Than Never: Workforce Supply Implications of Later Entry into Nursing. *Health Affairs*, 26(1), 178–185.

Baggs, J. G. (1989). Intensive Care Unit Use and Collaboration Between Nurses and Physicians. *Heart and Lung*, *18*, 332–338.

Baggs, J. G., Schmitt, M. H., Mushlin, A., Mitchell, P. H., Eldredge, D. H., Oakes, D., et al. (1999). Association Between Nurse-Physician Collaboration and Patient Outcomes in Three Intensive Care Units. *Critical Care Medicine*, 27(9), 1991–1998.

Benjamin, J. (1988). *The Bonds of Love: Psychoanalysis, Feminism, & the Problem of Domination*. New York: Pantheon Books.

Benner, P. (1984). *From Novice to Expert: Excellence and Power in Clinical Nursing Practice*. Menlo Park, CA: Addison-Wesley.

Benner, P. (1994). The Role of Articulation in Understanding Practice and Experience as Sources of Knowledge in Clinical Nursing. In J. Tully (Ed.), *Philosophy in an Age of Pluralism: The Philosophy of Charles Taylor in Question* (pp. 136–155). New York: Cambridge University Press.

Benner, P. (2000). The Roles of Embodiment, Emotion and Lifeworld for Rationality and Agency in Nursing Practice. *Nursing Philosophy*, *1*(1), 5–19.

Benner, P. (2005). Using the Dreyfus Model of Skill Acquisition to Describe and Interpret Skill Acquisition and Clinical Judgment in Nursing Practice and Education. *Bulletin of Science, Technology and Science Special Issue: Human Expertise in the Age of the Computer*, 24(3), 188–199.

Benner, P., Hooper-Kyriakidis, P., & Stannard, D. (1999). *Clinical Wisdom and Interventions in Critical Care: a Thinking-in-Action Approach*. Philadelphia: Saunders.

Benner, P., & Sullivan, W. (2005). Current Controversies in Clinical Care: Challenges to Professionalism—Work Integrity and the Call to Renew and Strengthen the Social Contract of the Professions. *American Journal of Critical Care*, 14(1), 78.

Benner, P., Tanner, C., & Chesla, C. (2009). *Expertise in Nursing Practice: Caring Clinical Judgment and Ethics* (2nd ed.). New York: Springer.

Benner, P., & Wrubel, J. (1982). Skilled Clinical Knowledge: The Value of Perceptual Awareness. *Nursing Educator*, 7(3), 11–17.

Benner, P., & Wrubel, J. (1989). *The Primacy of Caring: Stress and Coping in Health and Illness*. Menlo Park, CA: Addison-Wesley.

Berlin, L., & Sechrist, K. (2002). The Shortage of Doctorally Prepared Nursing Faculty: A Dire Situation. *Nursing Outlook*, 50(2), 50–56.

Bloom, B. S. (1968). *Taxonomy of Educational Objectives: The Classification of Educational Goals by a Committee of College and University Examiners*. New York: McKay.

Borgmann, A. (1984). *Technology and the Character of Contemporary Life: A Philosophical Inquiry.* Chicago: University of Chicago Press.

Bourdieu, P. (1990). *The Logic of Practice* (R. Nice, Trans.). Palo Alto, CA: Stanford University Press.

Boyer, E. L. (1990). *Scholarship Reconsidered: Priorities of the Professoriate.* San Francisco: Jossey-Bass.

Bowker, G. C., & Star, S. L. (1999). *Sorting Things Out: Classification and Its Consequences.* Cambridge, MA: MIT Press.

Brannan, J., White, A., & Bezanson, J. (2008). Simulator Effects on Cognitive Skills and Confidence Levels. *Journal of Nursing Education, 47*(11), 495–500.

Brown, E. (1948). *Nursing for the Future, A. Report Prepared for the National Nursing Council.* New York: Russell Sage Foundation.

Buerhaus, P. I., Donelan, K., Ulrich, B. T., Norman, L., & Dittus, R. (2006). State of the Registered Nurse Workforce in the United States. *Nursing Economics, 24*(1), 6–12, 13.

Buerhaus, P. I., Donelan, K., Ulrich, B. T., DesRoches, C., & Dittus, R. (2007a). Trends in the Experiences of Hospital-Employed Registered Nurses: Results from Three National Surveys. *Nursing Economics, 25*(2), 69–80.

Buerhaus, P. I., Donelan, K., Ulrich, B. T., Norman, L., DesRoches, C., & Dittus, R. (2007b). Impact of the Nurse Shortage on Hospital Patient Care: Comparative Perspectives. *Health Affairs, 26*(3), 853–862.

Canadian Nurses' Association. Joint Position Statement, Promoting Continuing Competence for Registered Nurses. Retrieved March 25, 2009, from http://www.cna-aiic.ca/CNA/documents/pdf/publications/PS77_promoting_compe tence_e.pdf.

Carroll, T. L. (2007). SBAR and Nurse-Physician Communication: Pilot Testing an Education Intervention. *Nursing Administration Quarterly, 30*(3), 295–299.

Chan, G. K. (2005). Understanding End-of-Life Caring Practices in the Emergency Department: Developing Merleau-Ponty's Notions of Intentional Arc and Maximum Grip Through Praxis and Phronesis. *Journal of Nursing Philosophy, 6*(1), 19–32.

Chao, S., Anderson, K., & Hernandez, L. (2009). *IOM Workshop Report: Toward Health Equity and Patient-Centeredness Integrating Health Literacy, Disparities Reduction and Quality Improvement.* Washington, DC: National Academy Press.

Cheung, R., & Aiken, L. (2006). Hospital Initiatives to Support a Better-Educated Workforce. *Journal of Nursing Administration, 36*(7), 357–362.

Cooke, M., Irby, D., & O'Brien, B. (forthcoming). *Educating Doctors.* San Francisco: Jossey-Bass.

Cossentino, J. (2005). Ritualizing Expertise: A Non-Montessorian view of the Montessori Method. *American Journal of Education, 111*(2), 211–244.

Cronenwett, L., Sherwood, G., Barnsteiner, J., Disch, J., Johnson, J., Mitchell, P., et al. (2007). Quality and Safety Education for Nurses. *Nursing Outlook, 55*(3), 122–131.

Damasio, A. (1994). *Descartes' Error: Emotion, Reason and the Human Brain*. New York: Putnam.

Day, L. (2005). Current Controversies in Critical Care: Nursing Practice and Civic Professionalism. *American Journal of Critical Care, 14*(5), 434–437.

Dewey, J. (1933). *How We Think: A Restatement of the Relation of Reflective Thinking to the Educative Process*. Boston: Heath.

Dewey, J. (1987). *Experience and Nature*. Chicago: Open Court Press. (Originally published in 1925.)

Diekelmann, N., & Smythe, E. (2004). Covering Content and the Additive Curriculum: How Can I Use My Time with Students to Best Help Them Learn What They Need to Know? *Journal of Nursing Education, 43*(8), 341–345.

Dohm, A., & Shniper, L. (2007). Bureau of Labor Statistics: Employment Outlook: 2006–2016, Occupational Employment Projections to 2016. *Monthly Labor Review, 86,* 89.

Dreyfus, H. L. (1992). *What Computers Still Can't Do: A Critique of Artificial Reason*. Cambridge, MA: MIT Press.

Dreyfus, H., & Dreyfus, S. E. (1986). *Mind over Machine: The Power of Human Intuition and Expertise in the Era of the Computer*. New York: Free Press.

Dreyfus, H., Dreyfus, S., & Benner, P. (2009). Implications of the Phenomenology of Expertise for Teaching and Learning Everyday Skillful Ethical Comportment. In P. Benner & C. Tanner (Eds.), *Expertise in Nursing Practice, Caring Clinical Judgment and Ethics* (2nd ed., pp. 309–333). New York: Springer.

Dunne, J. (1993). *Back to the Rough Ground: "Phronesis" and "Techne" in Modern Philosophy and in Aristotle*. Notre Dame, IN: Notre Dame University Press.

Dunne, J. (1997). *Back to the Rough Ground: Practical Judgment and the Lure of Technique*. Notre Dame, IN: University of Notre Dame Press.

Eraut, M. (1994). *Developing Professional Knowledge and Competence*. Washington, DC: Falmer Press.

Estabrooks, C., Midodzi, W., Cummings, G., Ricker, K., & Giovannetti, P. (2005). The Impact of Hospital Nursing Characteristics on 30-Day Mortality. *Nursing Research, 54*(2), 74–84.

Folkman, S., & Lazarus, R. (1982). *A Transactional View of Stress and Coping*. New York: Springer.

Foster, C. R., Dahill, L. E., Golemon, L. A., & Tolentino, B. W. (2005). *Educating Clergy: Teaching Practices and Pastoral Imagination*. San Francisco: Jossey-Bass.

Fox, M. (2007). *Start with Medical Training to Fix US Health Care: CDC Head* [electronic version]. Retrieved 10/19/2007 from http://www.reuters.com/article/domesticNews/idUSN1428524820070714.

Freidson, E. (1970). *Professional Dominance: The Social Structure of Medical Care*. New York: Atherton Press.

Gadamer, H. G. (1975). *Truth and Method* (G. Barden & J. Cumming,Trans., 2nd ed.). London: Sheed and Ward.

Golde, C., & Walker, G. (Eds.). (2006). *Envisioning the Future of Doctoral Education: Preparing Stewards of the Discipline—Carnegie Essays on the Doctorate*. San Francisco: Jossey-Bass.

Greiner, A. C., & Knebel, E. (Eds.). (2003). *Health Professions Education: A Bridge to Quality*. Washington, DC: National Academy Press.

Grusec, J. E., & Hastings, P. D. (2007). *Handbook of Socialization: Theory and Research*. New York: Guilford Press.

Hatch, T. (2005). *Into the Classroom: Developing the Scholarship of Teaching and Learning*. San Francisco: Jossey-Bass.

Health Resources and Services Administration/Bureau of Health Professions. (2006). What Is Behind HRSA's Projected Supply, Demand, and Shortage of Registered Nurses? Retrieved March 25, 2009, from http://bhpr.hrsa.gov/healthworkforce/reports/behindrnprojections/2.htm, http://bhpr.hrsa.gov/healthworkforce/reports/behindrnprojections/3.htm.

Health Resources and Services Administration/Bureau of Health Professions. (2007). *The Registered Nurse Population: Findings from the 2004 National Sample Survey of Registered Nurses*. U. S. Department of Health and Human Services.

Huber, M. T., & Hutchings, P. (2005). *The Advancement of Learning: Building the Teaching Commons*. San Francisco: Jossey-Bass.

Institute of Medicine. (1983). *Personal Needs and Training for Biomedical and Behavioral Research*. Washington, DC: National Academy Press.

Institute of Medicine. (2008). *IOM Report: Evidence-Based Medicine and the Changing Nature of Healthcare: Workshop Summary*. Washington, DC: National Academy Press.

Ironside, P. M. (2004). "Covering Content" and Teaching Thinking: Deconstructing the Additive Curriculum. *Journal of Nursing Education*, 43(1), 5–12.

Ironside, P. M. (2008). Safeguarding Patients Through Continuing Competency. *Journal of Continuing Education in Nursing*, 39(2), 86–91.

Johnson, J. H. (1988). Differences in the Performance of Baccalaureate, Associate Degree, and Diploma Nurses: A Meta-Analysis. *Research in Nursing & Health, 11*(3), 183–197.

Jonsen, A. R., Siegler, M., & Winslade, W. J. (2002). *Clinical Ethics* (5th ed.). New York: Appleton & Lange.

Kerdeman, D. (2004). Pulled Up Short: Challenging Self-Understanding as a Focus of Teaching and Learning. In J. Dunne & P. Hogan (Eds.), *Education and Practice: Upholding the Integrity of Teaching and Learning* (pp. 144–158). London: Blackwell.

Kjervik, D. K. (2006). Creation of the National Institute of Nursing Research: Talking the Walk for Nursing Research. *Journal of Professional Nursing, 22*(1), 4–5.

Kohn, L. T., Corrigan, J. M., & Donaldson, M. S. (Eds.). (2000). *To Err Is Human: Building a Safer Health System*. Washington, DC: National Academy Press.

Landeen, J., & Jeffries, P. (2008). Focus on Simulation—Integrating Simulation into Teaching Practice. *Journal of Nursing Education, 47*(11), 487–488.

Lasater, K., & Nielson, A. (2009). Educational Innovations: Reflective Journaling for Clinical Judgment Development and Evaluation. *Journal of Nursing Education, 48*(1), 36–39.

Lave, J., & Wenger, E. (1991). *Situated Learning: Legitimate Peripheral Participation*. New York: Cambridge University Press.

Leape, L. L. (1994). Error in Medicine. *Journal of the American Medical Association, 272*(23), 1851–1857.

Logstrup, K. E. (1995). *Metaphysics, I.* Milwaukee: Marquette University Press.

Lutz, S., & Root, D. (2007). Nurses, Consumer Satisfaction, and Pay for Performance. *Healthcare Financial Management, 61*(10), 56–63.

Lysaught, J. P. (1970). *An Abstract for Action*. New York: McGraw-Hill.

Mahaffey, E. (2002). The Relevance of Associate Degree Nursing Education: Past, Present, Future. *Online Journal of Issues in Nursing, 7*(2).

Malloch, K., & Porter-O'Grady, T. (Eds.). (2006). *An Introduction to Evidence-Based Practice for Nursing and Healthcare*. Sudbury: Jones and Bartlett.

Meleis, A. I. (2006). *Theoretical Nursing: Development and Progress* (4th ed.). Philadelphia: J. B. Lippincott.

Merleau-Ponty, M. (1962). *Phenomenology of Perception* (C. Smith, Trans.). New York: Humanities Press.

Mohrmann, M. E. (2006). On Being True to Form. In C. Taylor & R. Dell'Oro (Eds.), *Health and Human Flourishing: Religion, Medicine, and Moral Anthropology* (pp. 90–102). Washington, DC: Georgetown University Press.

My Jewish Learning. (n.d.). Retrieved March 21, 2009, from http://www.myjewishlearning.com/practices/Ethics/Caring_For_Others/Tikkun_Olam_Repairing_the_World_.shtml.

National Council of State Boards of Nursing. (2005). Meeting the Ongoing Challenge of Continued Competence. https://www.ncsbn.org/Continued_Comp_Paper_TestingServices.pdf. Retrieved March 25, 2009.

National League for Nursing. (2006). *Nursing Data Review, Academic Year 2004–2005, Baccalaureate, Associate Degree, and Diploma Programs.* New York: National League for Nursing.

Nelson, S. (2006). Ethical Expertise and the Problem of the Good Nurse. In S. Nelson & S. Gordon (Eds.), *The Complexities of Care: Nursing Reconsidered.* Ithaca, NY: Cornell University Press.

NHLBI ARDS Network. (2004). Retrieved March 31, 2009, from http://www.ardsnet.org/.

Orsolini-Hain, L. M. (2008). *An Interpretive Phenomenological Study on the Influences on Associate Degree Prepared Nurses to Return to School to Earn a Higher Degree in Nursing.* San Francisco: University of California, San Francisco.

Page, A. (Ed.). (2004). *Keeping Patients Safe: Transforming the Work Environment of Nurses.* Washington, DC: Institute of Medicine National Academy Press.

Pope, B. B., Rodzen, L., & Spross, G. (2008). Raising the SBAR: How Better Communication Improves Patient Outcomes. *Nursing and Health Care Perspectives, 38*(3), 41–43.

Porter-O'Grady, T., & Malloch, K. (2003). Nurses as Knowledge Workers. *Creative Nursing, 9*(2), 6–9.

Porter-O'Grady, T., & Malloch, K. (2007). *Quantum Leadership A Resource for Health Care* (2nd ed.). Sudbury, MA: Jones and Bartlett.

PricewaterhouseCoopers' Health Research Institute. (2007). *What Works: Healing the Healthcare Staffing Shortage.* Retrieved 2009, from http://pwchealth.com/cgi-local/hcregister.cgi?link=reg/pubwhatworks.pdf.

Robert Wood Johnson Foundation. (2007). *Facts and Controversies About Nurse Staffing Policy: A Look at Existing Models, Enforcement Issues, and Research Needs.* http://www.rwjf.org/files/research/nursingissue5revfinal.pdf.

Rodriguez, L. (2007). *Confronting Life and Death Responsibility: The Lived Experiences of Nursing Students and Nursing Faculty Response to Practice Breakdown and Errors in Nursing School.* San Francisco: University of California.

Rubin, J. (2009). Impediments to the Development of Clinical Knowledge and Ethical Judgment in Critical Care Nursing. In P. Benner, C. Tanner, & C. Chesla (Eds.), *Expertise in Nursing Practice: Caring, Clinical Judgment, and Ethics* (pp. 171–198). New York: Springer.

Ruddick, S. (1989). *Maternal Thinking: Toward a Politics of Peace*. Boston: Beacon Press.

Saad, L. (2006). *Nurses Top List of Most Honest and Ethical Professions*. Retrieved April 28, 2008, from http://www.calnurses.org/media-center/in-the-news/2006/december/page.jsp?itemID=29117737.

Sagara, M. (2003). *Japanese Children's Concept of Death*. San Francisco: University of California.

SBAR Technique for Communication: A Situational Briefing Model. (2007). *Institute for Healthcare Improvement*. Retrieved October 29, 2008, from http://www.ihi.org/IHI/Topics/PatientSafety/SafetyGeneral/Tools/SBAR TechniqueforCommunicationASituationalBriefingModel.htm.

Schön, D. A. (1987). *Educating the Reflective Practitioner: Toward a New Design for Teaching and Learning in the Professions*. San Francisco: Jossey-Bass.

Seropian, M. A., Brown, K., Gavilanes, J. S., & Driggers, B. (2004a). Simulation: Not Just a Manikin. *Journal of Nursing Education, 43*(4), 164–169.

Seropian, M., Brown, K., Gavilanes, J., & Driggers, B. (2004b). An Approach to Simulation Program Development. *Journal of Nursing Education, 43*(4), 170–174.

Sheppard, S. D., Macatangay, K., Colby, A., Sullivan, W. M., & Shulman, L. S. (2008). *Educating Engineers: Designing for the Future of the Field*. San Francisco: Jossey-Bass.

Shulman, L. S., & Wilson, S. M. (2004). *The Wisdom of Practice: Essays on Teaching, Learning, and Learning to Teach*. San Francisco: Jossey-Bass.

Smedley, B. D., Stith, A. Y., & Nelson, A. R. (Eds.). (2003). *Unequal Treatment: Confronting Racial and Ethnic Disparities in Health Care*. Washington, DC: National Academies Press.

Sullivan, W. (2004). *Work and Integrity: The Crisis and Promise of Professionalism in America* (2nd ed.). San Francisco: Jossey-Bass.

Sullivan, W. (2005). Challenges to Professionalism: Work Integrity and the Call to Renew and Strengthen the Social Contract of the Professions. *American Journal of Critical Care, 14*(1), 78–80, 84.

Sullivan, W., Colby, A., Wegner, J., Bond, L., & Shulman, L. (2007). *Educating Lawyers: Preparation for the Profession of Law*. San Francisco: Jossey-Bass.

Sullivan, W., & Rosin, M. (2008). *A New Agenda for Higher Education: Shaping a Life of the Mind for Practice*. San Francisco: Jossey-Bass.

Swankin, D., LeBuhn, R., & Morrison, R. (2006). *Implementing Continuing Competency Requirements for Health Care Professionals*. Washington, DC: AARP. http://www.cacenter.org/Implementing%20Continuing%20Comp etency%20Requirements%20for%20Health%20Care%20Practitioners% 20-%202006.pdf.

Tammelleo, A. D. (2001). Failure to Keep Physicians Informed—Death Results. *Nursing Law's Regan Report*, 41(11), 2.

Tammelleo, A. D. (2002). Nurses Failed to Advocate for Their Patient. *Nursing Law's Regan Report*, 42(8), 2.

Tanner, C. A. (1998). Curriculum for the 21st Century—Or Is It the 21-Year Curriculum? *Journal of Nursing Education*, 37(9), 383–384.

Tanner, C. A. (2004). The Meaning of Curriculum: Content to Be Covered or Stories to Be Heard? *Journal of Nursing Education*, 43(1), 3–4.

Taylor, C. (1985a). Social Theory as Practice. In C. Taylor (Ed.), *Philosophical Papers* (Vol. 1, pp. 42–57). Cambridge: Cambridge University Press.

Taylor, C. (1985b). What Is Human Agency? In C. Taylor (Ed.), *Philosophical Papers* (Vol. 1, pp. 15–44). Cambridge: Cambridge University Press.

Taylor, C. (1985c). The Concept of a Person. In *Human Agency and Language: Philosophical Papers, Vol. 1* (pp. 97–114). Cambridge, UK: Cambridge university Press.

Taylor, C. (1993). Explanation and Practical Reason. In M. Nussbaum & A. Sen (Eds.), *The Quality of Life* (pp. 208–231). Oxford: Clarendon Press.

Taylor, C. (2007). *A Secular Age*. Cambridge, MA: Harvard University Press.

Thomas, L. (1995). *The Youngest Science: Notes of a Medicine-Watcher*. New York: Penguin Press.

Thompson, T., & Bonnel, W. (2008). A Unique Simulation Teaching Method. *Journal of Nursing Education*, 47(11), 524–527.

Tilley, D. (2008). Competency in Nursing: A Concept Analysis. *Journal of Continuing Nursing Education*, 39(2), 58–64.

U.S. Department of Health and Human Services. (2004). *The Registered Nurse Population: National Sample Survey of Registered Nurses*. Retrieved April 1, 2009, from http://www.hrsa.gov.

Walker, G., Golde, C., Jones, L., Bueschel, A., & Hutchings, P. (2008). *The Formation of Scholars: Rethinking Doctoral Education for the Twenty-First Century*. San Francisco: Jossey-Bass.

Weick, K. E., & Sutcliffe, K. M. (2001). *Managing the Unexpected: Assuring High Performance in an Age of Complexity*. San Francisco: Jossey-Bass.

Weiss, S. (1992). Measurement of the Sensory Qualities in Tactile Interaction. *Journal of Nursing Research*, 41(2), 82–86.

Whitbeck, C. (1983). A Different Reality: Feminist Ontology. In C. Gould (Ed.), *Beyond Domination, New Perspectives on Women and Philosophy* (pp. 64–88). Totowa, NJ: Rowman & Allenheld.

Williams, B. (2001). Developing Critical Reflection for Professional Practice Through Problem-Based Learning. *Journal of Advanced Nursing*, 34(1), 27–34.

Wong, F., Kam, Y., Cheung, S., Chung, L., Chan, K., Chan, A., et al. (2008). Framework for Adopting a Problem-Based Learning Approach in a Simulated Clinical Setting. *Journal of Nursing Education, 47*(11), 508–514.

Wuthnow, R. (1993). *Acts of Compassion, Caring for Others and Helping Ourselves*. Princeton, NJ: Princeton University Press.

Yuan, H., Williams, B., & Fan, L. (2008). A Systematic Review of Selected Evidence on Developing Nursing Students' Critical Thinking Through Problem-Based Learning. *Nurse Education Today, 28*(6), 657–663.

INDEX